Welcome to

THE

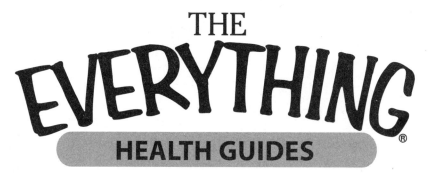

When you're faced with a pressing health issue, your first instinct is to find out as much about it as you can. With so much conflicting information out there, where can you turn for professional, supportive advice?

Packed with the most recent, up-to-date data, THE EVERYTHING® HEALTH GUIDES help ensure that you get a good diagnosis, choose the best doctor, and find the right medical treatment. With this one comprehensive resource, you and your family members have all the information you could possibly need—at your fingertips.

THE EVERYTHING® HEALTH GUIDES are an extension of the bestselling Everything® series in the health category, which also includes *The Everything® Diabetes Book* and *The Everything® Menopause Book*. Accessible and easy to read, THE EVERYTHING® HEALTH GUIDES provide specific details and clear examples that relate to your given medical situation. If you're looking for one-stop, all-inclusive guides that allow you to understand and become more in tune with your body, this groundbreaking series is the perfect tool for you.

Visit the entire Everything® series at *www.everything.com*

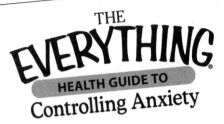

THE EVERYTHING® HEALTH GUIDE TO
Controlling Anxiety

Dear Reader,

As a psychotherapist specializing in anxiety disorders I have spent the past fifteen years treating hundreds of adults, adolescents, and children suffering from various anxiety problems. My education, training, and experience as a mental health clinician have given me the ability to help many clients overcome anxiety and go on to lead full and rewarding lives. But I think it was my own struggle with anxiety and panic that enabled me to connect and work so well with anxious clients. Beyond all the school and training, I know how it feels. Performance anxiety tripped me up over my lifetime in public speaking, on tennis courts, and in horse shows. Panic attacks on airplanes grounded me for years. By seeking treatment, both conventional and alternative, I took control of my anxiety, which ever so slowly lost its power and hold over me.

My struggle with anxiety continues, but it doesn't stop me from doing things anymore. Writing this book caused me to feel anxious and panicky at times, but I have developed methods of overcoming these feelings and continuing on toward my goals. This is what I wish to impart to you; anxiety is uncomfortable and difficult, but it's also common and manageable. Use this book as a resource and guide as you begin your battle with anxiety and take control of your life.

Best Wishes,

Diane Peters Mayer

THE
EVERYTHING

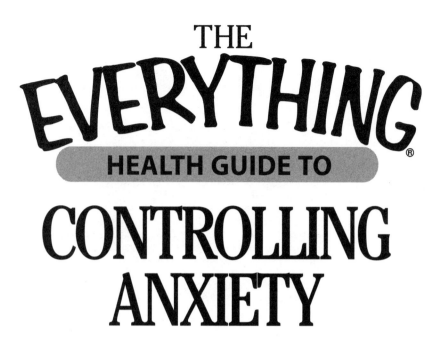

HEALTH GUIDE TO

CONTROLLING
ANXIETY

Professional advice to get you
through any situation

Diane Peters Mayer, M.S.W.

Adams Media
Avon, Massachusetts

Dedication

To those dear readers who suffer from
anxiety and their loved ones—this book is for you.

• • •

Publishing Director: Gary M. Krebs
Associate Managing Editor: Laura M. Daly
Associate Copy Chief: Brett Palana-Shanahan
Acquisitions Editor: Kate Burgo
Development Editor: Katie McDonough
Associate Production Editor: Casey Ebert
Technical Reviewer: John DeRosalia, L.C.S.W.

Director of Manufacturing: Susan Beale
Associate Director of Production: Michelle Roy Kelly
Cover Design: Paul Beatrice, Matt LeBlanc
Layout and Graphics: Colleen Cunningham,
Holly Curtis, Erin Dawson, Sorae Lee

An Everything® Series Book.
Everything® and everything.com® are registered trademarks of F+W Publications, Inc.

Published by Adams Media, an F+W Publications Company
57 Littlefield Street, Avon, MA 02322 U.S.A.
www.adamsmedia.com

ISBN: 1-59337-429-1

Printed in the United States of America.

J I H G F E D C B A

Library of Congress Cataloging-in-Publication Data
Peters Mayer, Diane.
The Everything health guide to controlling anxiety / author, Diane Peters Mayer.
p. cm. -- (An everything series book)
ISBN 1-59337-429-1
1. Anxiety--Popular works. 2. Anxiety--Treatment--Popular works. I. Title. II. Series: Everything series.

RC531.P42 2005
616.85'2206--dc22

2005015475

This publication is designed to provide accurate and authoritative information with regard to the subject matter covered. It is sold with the understanding that the publisher is not engaged in rendering legal, accounting, or other professional advice. If legal advice or other expert assistance is required, the services of a competent professional person should be sought.

—From a *Declaration of Principles* jointly adopted by a Committee of the American Bar Association and a Committee of Publishers and Associations

Many of the designations used by manufacturers and sellers to distinguish their products are claimed as trademarks. Where those designations appear in this book and Adams Media was aware of a trademark claim, the designations have been printed with initial capital letters.

All the examples and dialogues used in this book are fictional and have been created by the author to illustrate disciplinary situations.

Acknowledgments

• • •

Thanks to my agent Jacky Sach, and to everyone at Adams Media. My appreciation also goes out to Dr. David Nover, Dr. Barbara Gazze, Dr. Frank Dattilio, and Dr. Jonathan Warren for giving me their time and expertise. As always, thanks to my family, who continue to support me in my writing endeavors.

Contents

Top Ten Ways to Begin Controlling Anxiety

1. See your physician for a complete medical checkup.

2. Educate yourself about anxiety, its disorders, causes, and treatments.

3. Go to a mental health specialist for an evaluation and treatment.

4. Become proactive in your treatment planning and recovery.

5. Learn how to manage stress and control chronic worry.

6. Eat whole foods, avoid processed foods, sugars, and fats, and drink plenty of water.

7. Exercise regularly.

8. Eliminate substances like alcohol, caffeine, nicotine, and illegal drugs from your life.

9. Find exercises and techniques that will help you relax mentally and physically.

10. Learn to enjoy life, connect with family and friends, and make leisure time for yourself.

Introduction

Everyone experiences anxiety. Stressful situations make up a good portion of the day for most people. If you have to get your kids off to school every morning or have a daily commute on traffic-choked highways, you probably feel anxious during these times. Maybe you became anxious when you had to take a test in school and still do when you give a weekly report to your boss. Major life transitions, such as graduating from high school or college, or getting married or divorced, or experiencing the death of a loved one will cause extreme anxiety that can last for long periods of time.

Anxiety is part of living, of being human, and is an important component of your ability to set goals, perform at your best, and achieve what you put your mind to. Anxiety is also a warning mechanism telling you that things are not right or dangerous, propelling you to take action to protect yourself. In fact, without anxiety humankind would never have survived. It is a normal reaction to life situations that are unpleasant, sad, or scary.

General, manageable anxiety happens to everyone, but anxiety becomes a problem when it turns into a disruptive chronic condition that hinders how you function in daily life. Anxiety disorders are the most common mental health problem in the United States, and approximately 20 million adults, adolescents, and children have been diagnosed with an anxiety disorder. Disorders include panic disorders, social phobia, and stress disorders. Whether you or a family member develops an anxiety disorder depends on any number of related factors, such as heredity, life experiences, and coping skills.

If you or a loved one has been diagnosed with an anxiety disorder there are many conventional and alternative treatments that can help ease acute symptoms and set you on the path to healing and recovery. The most important elements in controlling anxiety include awareness, education, getting professional help, treatment, and reaching out for support. It can be intimidating and difficult to admit that you are having significant problems functioning in your daily life, but not getting help can lead to a chronic condition and years of suffering.

Anxiety disorders are often misunderstood and many people think you should be able to overcome symptoms of anxiety by sheer willpower. If you have an anxiety disorder you know this is untrue. This book includes information about anxiety and its disorders, conventional treatments as well as alternative therapies, and how changing your lifestyle can go a long way to vastly improving the way you feel. You'll also find resources and information on the latest research and self-help exercises and techniques to set you on your way to recovery.

Often the hardest part of getting control of your anxiety is recognizing that you have a problem and that you need help. In picking up this book, you've already done that, so you're well on your way. Just stick with it, be optimistic, and read on—help is only a few pages away.

CHAPTER 1

Anxiety: The Basics

Anxiety is both a positive and negative force in humans. On the one hand, it protects and adds vitality to one's life, but when it goes out of control it can negatively disrupt daily function. Anxiety is a complex issue, so the best way to start learning about it is to obtain some basic information, discover the history of anxiety, and find out how the mental health community classifies anxiety disorders.

A Human Quality

Anxiety is an innate quality of being a human being. From humans' early stone-age ancestors to modern humankind, anxiety is one of your most important defense mechanisms. Without it you would not be able to sense danger and protect yourself. Anxiety is a normal response to certain life situations; it's totally natural to feel anxious about losing your job or to worry when you learn a hurricane is headed your way.

Though anxiety has a negative connotation, it does have a positive side. It's important to understand that if anxiety was absent from the human condition, then absent too would be the passion, vitality, and zest that make life worth living. The key is to think of anxiety as your own energy and express it in meaningful, productive ways. How you view anxiety and learn from it makes all the difference. As the saying goes, "attitude is everything."

Anxiety, like physical pain, tells you that something is wrong. It can spark the awareness and understanding that leads to solutions to make necessary life changes. Anxiety can encourage you to achieve your personal best, to attain goals, and to reach for your dreams, if you learn how to use it constructively. But if anxiety becomes painful, acute, and persistent and turns into a chronic condition that wreaks psychological, physiological, and behavioral havoc, it becomes impossible to function normally and enjoy life. When that happens, anxiety becomes a disorder.

Defining Anxiety

Anxiety is defined as a state of intense apprehension, agitation, tension, and dread arising from a real or perceived threat of imminent danger. It affects both mind and body with a host of symptoms that can negatively impact mental and physical health. Though it is an experience unique to each person, anxiety has general characteristics that include increased heart rate, muscle tension, shallow breathing, trembling, sweating, and worry or feelings of unease.

Anxiety symptoms can be mild to severe and can become so disturbing that people often seek immediate relief by either departing the scene or avoiding stressful situations. Other conditions, such as depression and substance abuse, are often associated with anxiety. While some milder forms of anxiety can be managed through simple relaxation techniques and lifestyle changes, managing the more severe forms of anxiety often requires medical treatment.

Am I Going Crazy?

Many people fear they are going insane while experiencing some form of anxiety, as the symptoms are often acute and intense. Senses and perceptions may become distorted; for example, you may experience tunnel vision or the sensation of being outside your own body. These sensations are frightening. Some fear they will "freak out" and hurt loved ones. Feeling totally out of control is certainly uncomfortable, but it does not mean you're crazy. Consider the following case example:

> Cheryl suffered from daily panic attacks for years. When an attack came on she feared she was going crazy. Her senses were off, she felt out of her body, normal house noises like the dishwasher

became earsplitting, or she heard buzzing in her head. She felt that she had no control over her reactions and behaviors and feared that she was going insane. Her greatest fears were the thoughts that played over and over again that she would kill her husband.

Is Cheryl insane? No. Does she really want to kill her husband? Absolutely not. Cheryl manages to take care of her children and work part-time, but she suffers from panic disorder. Her symptoms are severe and her thoughts are so bizarre and frightening that she firmly believes she is losing her mind. She isn't—she just needs help.

Alert

The symptoms of anxiety are common to many life-threatening illnesses, such as heart disease and stroke. If you or anyone you know is experiencing even one of them, do not hesitate to seek medical attention immediately. Anxiety is not something to put off until the symptoms grab your attention by getting worse.

Is It All in My Head or Do I Have a Disease?

Many of the symptoms of anxiety disorders are in your head, including obsessive thoughts, chronic worry, and irrational fears that can make daily life miserable. But are the symptoms emotionally based, or is there an organic explanation? According to the majority of psychiatrists and mental health professionals today, anxiety disorders fit the definition of disease. This is because theories about the causes of anxiety have changed in recent years and now include possibilities such as chemical imbalances and even speculation that there is an anxiety gene.

But some mental health experts, such as Thomas Szasz, author of *The Myth of Mental Illness*, reject the disease theory for anxiety and other disorders that are without scientific evidence of physical impairment, claiming that behavior alone does not constitute a disease. Still others state that anxiety has internal characteristics, such as moods and feelings, that cannot be examined by hard science. Many theories exist, and experts in the field are unable to agree on the origins of anxiety disorders or how to treat them.

Some professionals believe that anxiety attacks, chronic worry, and other symptoms, indicate a biological disease. This could be caused by a biochemical imbalance, possibly in the brain's neurotransmitters. Some theorize that unconscious conflicts from childhood are the source of the anxiety, or that internal and external struggles are creating the anxiety. Various learning theories posit that anxiety is a learned behavior from childhood. Many experts agree that stress and trauma set the stage for anxiety disorders, and still others believe that anxiety is caused by a combination of biological, psychological, and social factors.

What Is a Disorder?

A psychological disorder is a mental disturbance of thought or emotion that impairs "normal" functioning and creates psychic distress. Though the terms mental disorder and mental illness are used interchangeably, disorder is a much less alarming term than illness. The term mental illness can convey images of being "sick" or "crazy." Also, some experts believe that using the word disorder evades the questions over the biological basis for conditions like anxiety.

Classified mental disorders range from mild distress, to the more severe anxiety disorders, to conditions that cause the individual to diverge from reality. Anxiety disorders can be grievous and disabling, and though the individuals who suffer from them may feel like they are going crazy, they are not. The anxiety sufferer is grounded in reality and does not split off into an unreal world. Read the following cases to find the distinctions:

> *Mark, who is in his thirties, has had a phobia toward snakes since he was five years old. When he was a child, his parents took him camping, and while walking in the woods with his mother, he startled a snake, which slithered away. His mother was afraid of snakes so she began to scream, which frightened Mark. Since that time, whenever*

Mark sees a snake, he becomes paralyzed with fear, feels like throwing up, and is unable to move until the snake leaves and the anxiety lessens. When he was younger even pictures of snakes would create panic, but that eased as he matured. However, his love of hiking and camping is severely curtailed because he fears he'll come across a snake again.

Rachel is a brilliant student. After high school she was accepted at an Ivy League college. From college she went right into law school. In the beginning of her last year, she began to exhibit strange behaviors, such as, withdrawing socially from friends, losing all interest in school, and had angry outbursts for no apparent reason. Her friends began to shy away from her, and her family believed it was the schoolwork overload that was making her anxious. But in the last semester, Rachel had a psychotic break and began having hallucinations. She heard voices coming from her wrist bone telling her what a bad girl she was, and that she should kill herself.

Mark has an anxiety disorder, a simple phobia. He is high-functioning in his day to day life, is fully in touch with reality, and though his phobia keeps him from enjoying activities he loves, it only affects a small part of his life. Rachel on the other hand, could no longer operate normally in the world. She became out of touch and lost her ability to think rationally. To her, the voices in her wrist bone were real, and she believed that what they said was true. Fearing that Rachel might hurt herself, her family had her institutionalized until she was stabilized.

Essential

Research indicates that there is a high incidence of suicide attempts in people with anxiety, due to the panic and distress common with these disorders. The suicide numbers for panic disorders are the highest among psychological disorders, and women are more likely to make an attempt than men, especially women who live alone.

Though anxiety disorders can totally disrupt and disable one's life, anxiety sufferers do not experience a break with the real world. And though symptoms like Cheryl's thoughts about killing her husband are strange and scary, she is aware how strange those thoughts are. This ability to recognize a problem is what distinguishes anxiety victims from those with severe mental conditions—and what makes their condition manageable.

Fear Versus Anxiety

In reference books fear is given as a synonym for anxiety. The words are commonly used interchangeably, but actually they have decidedly different meanings. Both are responses to a threat, but the difference is that fear is a reaction to something that is definable. It is being afraid of an external object or circumstance that can really harm you, that makes hearts pound and knees shake. But anxiety is not clearly defined. It is a perceived threat, a nameless internal worry, an accumulation of "what ifs" that haunt your imagination.

Consider this example. Joe is driving on a two-lane road. Suddenly, a car going in the opposite direction veers toward him. Joe reacts quickly, swerves, and avoids being hit. Heart pounding, Joe pulls over knowing he had a close call. Everything that happened to Joe can be expressed specifically and concretely. His body reacted to his fear, adrenaline and other stress hormones flooded his body, and he acted to avoid being hit. This experience won't stop Joe from driving again, but he will be more cautious, especially on that same stretch of road. Joe had a normal, fear-based reaction.

Now consider this second example. Jane is driving on a two-lane road. Suddenly, for no apparent reason, Jane begins to feel nervous. She feels a rush of heat course through her body, her heart begins to race and her head feels tight and begins to pound. Then her vision blurs. Jane is terrified of these sensations, turns her car around, and goes home. Over the next weeks, Jane has three other anxiety attacks on the same stretch of road and starts to avoid that road. But then she has attacks on other roads. Soon Jane begins to be afraid of driving altogether. She can't turn off the worry that the frightening feelings will appear, and that her vision will blur, making her crash her car. She's tried to stop thinking these thoughts, but that does not help. The only thing that makes her feel better is when she is in the safety of her home. Eventually, Jane limits her driving to no more than a mile from home. It is the unknown, the unexpected, and the possibility of disaster that makes the disturbing feelings of anxiety so difficult to cope with. Jane experiences anxiety associated with driving; this is not just fear.

Question

If you get nervous in traffic, does that mean you have an anxiety disorder?
Being "nervous" while driving in traffic does not mean you have an anxiety disorder. But, if your nervousness persists or worsens, you should be checked out by your family doctor or be seen by a mental health professional.

Anxiety in Ancient Cultures

Only as recently as 1980 did the American Psychiatric Association officially acknowledge anxiety disorder. Prior to this time, people who suffered from one of these disorders were dealt with in a variety of ways, from being locked up to being prayed for. From early civilization to our present culture, people suffering from mental disturbances have been seeking relief, and healers have created remedies based on the prevalent theories of the time.

It was universally believed by primitive civilizations that mental illness was caused by the supernatural: evil, magic, curses, and spells. The healers were medicine men, shamans, head priests, and tribal chiefs, who used charms, chanting, and dancing. However, in the historic progression of anxiety, magic and superstition were not limited to prehistoric man. These were actually believed to be the causes of anxiety and mental disorders centuries later.

⌐ Essential

The Hebrews' contribution to psychotherapy was the use of refocusing, a technique still used today to treat anxiety disorders, which held that people feeling mental distress should talk about their problems. The Hebrews also brought humanitarianism to health care. By A.D. 490, they had established a hospital in Jerusalem specifically for persons with mental illness.

Babylonians (Mid-2000-1700 B.C.)

The Babylonians, tucked away in areas of Mesopotamia, were one of the first organized civilizations. It is during their time that the Code of Hammurabi was inscribed into stone. This is one of the first written codes of law in human history—a compilation of some 300 laws covering all aspects of people's lives at the time. This artifact offers a fairly clear picture of what things were like back then.

In this society, the first physicians were priests, but lay physicians were also common. Babylonians practiced a form of animism, which is the belief that objects of nature and the universe possess souls and intelligence and are divine. Cures for disease were asked of religious and magical healers.

Egyptians

The Egyptians believed that disease was caused by supernatural powers. Imhotep, the Egyptian healer, was physician to the king. He became the "god of medicine," and his temple became a medical school and hospital. Their patients were treated with drugs and encouraged to occupy their time with cruises down the Nile, drawing and painting, and other activities of interest to them. Getting patients involved in outside activities and interests is an important method today in the treatment of anxiety and other mental disorders. But what sets Egypt apart from other ancient civilizations of that time was its recognition of emotional disorders. Temples called Serapeums were built, named after Serapis, the god of sleep. There patients would pray, purge, and use other methods to evoke certain dreams that they believed were healing and would solve their problems. After they awoke, priests would interpret the meanings of the dreams.

The Egyptians recognized anxiety disorders that the Greeks would later call *hysteria*—from the Greek *hysteron*, meaning uterus. The Egyptians believed that nervous symptoms constituted a female disease caused by incorrect positioning of the uterus. Healing was a fumigation procedure to bring the uterus back into normal position. Ingredients thought to have healing properties were burned, and the fumes were then entered vaginally. Though the treatment sounds odd, the Egyptians were on to something—today, more women report anxiety disorders and seek treatment than men.

Fact

Using sleep to heal emotional problems was a precursor to Freud's use of hypnosis and to the present theory and use of hypnotherapy. The interpretation of dreams led to one of the basics of Freudian psychoanalytic theory, that dreams were the path into the unconscious. Early Egyptian healers' interpretation of dreams was remarkable in its belief in the importance of the unconscious.

Greeks

The most significant contribution of ancient Greece in the history of medicine and mental disorders was the movement away from religious, supernatural causes of disease to rational beliefs, that is, natural phenomena. It began with Greek philosophers like Plato, Socrates, and Aristotle, whose teachings turned man's search for answers to his problems, from external causes to himself. The four elements, earth, air, water, and fire, were used to explain the world in physical terms. Hippocrates, called the "Father of Medicine," used these ideas to formulate his theory of disease, the four humors. Though his theory proved to be wrong, the idea that disease stems from natural causes was revolutionary. Hippocrates recorded the first classification of mental disorders, which included: mania, melancholia, and paranoia. He emphasized clinical medicine and was the first to recognize that the brain is the central organ.

Plato's contributions to modern psychiatry were significant. He saw the connection between mind and body, believing that the physical state of the body was manifested by psychological reasons. He thought the center of the person was the soul, and that two souls existed: the rational that ruled the person and the irrational made up of desires and drives. Plato made this distinction centuries before Freud introduced his theory of the id, ego, and superego.

Essential

Perhaps Hippocrates's most important contributions were the standards he set for doctors, still practiced today. By taking the Hippocratic oath, physicians promise to be honest with patients, to "do no harm," and to keep patient confidentiality. Hippocrates's rules have stood the test of time, being adopted by medical schools all over the world.

Romans (27 B.C.–A.D. 284)

Roman theories were less philosophical and more practical than the Greek philosophies that greatly influenced them. The central principle was that people could achieve happiness only by keeping themselves composed and untroubled by external events. If a person was "perturbed," he suffered from mental distress. Treatment for illness included prayer, herbal remedies, and serene surroundings. Two of the most important contributions of the Romans in treating mental disorders were beliefs that physical ailments could be the result of emotional distress, and that if one accepted and understood the root of their mental distress, then they were capable of changing it. These ideas are the basis for modern psychotherapy: that awareness of the psyche is the locus for change.

A Timeline

In addition to knowing which civilizations contributed to the history of anxiety study and treatment, it's also important to discover how the passage of time affected the phenomenon. From the middle ages to present day, study, treatment, and understanding of anxiety have evolved by leaps and bounds; however, many of the theories and techniques of the past are still used today.

The Middle Ages (A.D. 500–A.D.1300)

The toppling of the Roman Empire saw the collapse of the Roman and Greek belief in natural causes for disease and mental afflictions. The belief in magic, mysticism, and demonology returned, and Catholicism became the official religion. Theories of the causes of disease included: the four humors, magic and superstition, astrology, and punishment by God. Cures included: purging, bleeding, herbal remedies, prayer, and exorcism.

The Renaissance (1300s–1600s)

Beginning in the fourteenth century, there was renewed interest in Greek and Roman ideas. This signaled the end of the rigid beliefs of the Middle Ages with its emphasis on the supernatural. This was the beginning of the Renaissance, a time of intellectual freedom and great contributions to art, literature, science, and medicine. It was also a time of development of scientific methods, for example, the microscope was invented, as well as the study of the body by dissection. For the most part, anxiety was still treated with magic, including potions, astrology, palmistry, and suggestion.

Fact

The four humors were: blood, phlegm, yellow bile, and black bile. Blood was associated with a sanguine personality, a passionate person. A phlegmatic personality was said to be dull and sluggish. Yellow bile, was connected to a quickness to anger and a depressed personality was represented by black bile.

The humanist movement that arose at this time made a significant contribution to modern psychology. Theirs was a realistic view of the world and human nature, and unlike the theories of the Middle Ages, they believed that human emotions were dominant over intellect, and that man had free will, thus taking us into modern thought.

The Nineteenth and Twentieth Centuries

Sigmund Freud (1856–1939), along with such stalwarts as William James, trained with the most eminent neurologist of his time, Jean-Martin Charcot (1825–1893). Charcot's research in the area of hysteria drew Freud's interest. He studied both hypnotism and hysteria and with a colleague, Josef Breuer (1842–1925), offered the concept that hysteria was a condition caused by psychological trauma. In 1893 Freud and Breuer published their first paper on hysteria treated by psychoanalysis. Freud described "anxiety neurosis," which expanded his previous study by covering mild anxiety and panic attacks. Two years later they published *Studies in Hysteria*. The book comprised Breuer's history of a young woman he called "Anna O." Freud speculated that often anxiety and hysteria could be interpreted on the grounds of patients' repressed trauma and unconscious memories from childhood.

By the latter half of the 1890s, Freud and Breuer discovered that hysterical symptoms could be diminished and relieved when traumatic memories, and the feelings they had engendered, were put into words. This method of treatment became the basis of modern psychotherapy. Within the waning years of the century, Freud was in the process of revamping a number of his theories. As Freud's theories were undergoing revision, so too were the medical profession's views of Charcot. Eventually, hypnosis fell into the category of the occult and would not again be seriously considered as a major diagnostic tool.

Freud's continuing experimentation resulted in new methods of treatment, including free association, dream interpretation, and psychoanalysis. His work and that of other researchers led to the escalation of talk therapies, shock therapy, and psychosurgery. Before the mid-nineteenth century, researchers studied the more severe forms of mental illness, but Freud was interested in people who functioned though neurotic, thus separating the milder forms of mental illness like the anxiety disorders.

Fact

Freud suffered from anxiety, was given to "spells," and was treated for agoraphobia. When he lectured he was racked with nerves and he had panic attacks. At times his anxiety was so extreme he would faint while having dinner.

The Rise of Medication

Medicine unveiled important discoveries that changed the way people with mental disorders were viewed and treated. The mid-nineteenth century saw the discovery of sedatives such as chloral hydrate, bromine, and Seconal, and in the early 1900s amphetamines and barbiturates, which have been used to relieve anxiety, were introduced. The introduction of Librium and the benzodiazepine tranquilizers also occurred at this time. The research to find new medications and to reduce the negative side effects of those presently available is ongoing.

The stress of World War I produced an enormous number of psychiatric cases, men suffering from "shell shock," (now called posttraumatic stress disorder) and various other responses to fear and anxiety. During this period, a physiologist, Walter Cannon (1871–1945), coined the terms "fight or flight" and "stress." The beginning of World War II saw renewed research and medical practice in combat neuroses.

Post-WWII

In 1949, the National Institute of Mental Health (NIMH) was established. Behavioral therapy, which began in the 1950s, used imagery to gradually desensitize the patient to his fears; the Soviets experimented with Cranial Electrotherapy Stimulation (CES) to treat anxiety; research on the neural basis of emotion had all but ceased during the war but was in full swing again within five years of the war's end. In 1952, the American Psychiatric Association published the Diagnostic and Statistical Manual of Mental Disorders, popularly known as DSM-1, the standard guide for mental health professionals for diagnosing, setting up treatment plans, and aiding researchers.

In the 1960s, the positive response of mental disorders to medications sparked the growth of neuroscience, largely with NIMH's support. From then on psychopharmacology became big business, along with attempts made to hide the negligible or side effects of some trial medications. In 1963, Valium (diazepam) was approved for use. From 1969 on, it was the most prescribed drug in the United States for the next fourteen years.

The 1960s and 1970s were a mixed bag of chemical innovation. DSM-II was published, replacing the term "hysteria" with "conversion reaction." Continued research on stress led to the following conclusions:

- A lifetime of intense stress may accelerate old age.
- Social stress may cause high blood pressure.
- An adrenaline rush could cause panic attacks.
- Short-term stress can enhance the immune system.

Research showed that protracted stress resulted in the suppression of the immune system, and the end of the 1970s saw the inclusion of "posttraumatic stress disorder" (PTSD), included in DSM-III.

Anxiety Statistics

According to the NIMH, 13.3 percent or 19.1 million people in the United States suffer from anxiety disorders. It is the number one mental disorder in children, adolescents, and adults, and a study published in the *Journal of Clinical Psychiatry* stated that treating anxiety disorders costs a staggering $42 billion plus a year. Other negative effects are lost workplace productivity, and emotional pain and disruption in one's personal and professional life.

It is clear that different forms of anxiety affect men and women differently. The breakdown given by the NIMH for anxiety disorders affecting adult men and women are:

- *Generalized anxiety disorder*: 4 million; Twice as many women diagnosed than men.
- *Obsessive-compulsive disorder*: 3.3 million; Equal in men and women.
- *Panic disorder*: 2.4 million; Twice as many women diagnosed than men.
- *Posttraumatic stress disorder*: 5.2 million; More women diagnosed than men.
- *Social anxiety disorder*: 5.3 million; Equal in men and women.
- *Specific phobia*: 6.3 million; Twice as many women diagnosed than men.

It is estimated that approximately 10 percent of children and adolescents will at one time suffer from an anxiety disorder. Though children and adolescents can develop any of them, separation anxiety disorder and specific phobia are more commonly diagnosed in children, and panic disorder and social phobia in adolescents. In childhood, gender differences are not significant but by puberty girls are more likely to be affected by anxiety than boys.

The latest edition of the DSM-IV, published in 1994, lists over 300 disorders. Under Anxiety Disorders, the DSM-IV, lists eleven disorders:

- Panic disorder without agoraphobia
- Panic disorder with agoraphobia
- Agoraphobia without history of panic disorder
- Specific phobia
- Social phobia
- Obsessive-compulsive disorder
- Posttraumatic stress disorder
- Acute stress disorder

- Generalized anxiety disorder
- Anxiety disorder due to a general medical condition

Anxiety disorder NOS (not otherwise specified), the last classification, includes disorders that feature anxiety or phobic avoidance that do not meet the criteria for: anxiety disorder, adjustment disorder with anxiety, or adjustment disorder with mixed anxiety and depressed mood.

Anxiety and panic attacks appear in many other disorders, for example, depressive disorders, such as bipolar disorders; adjustment disorders, eating disorders, and pain disorder. The DSM is referred to as the "bible" of the mental health community, but it has its critics, who range from mental health providers, to people who have been patients in the mental health system. Some see strengths in the DSM as a guide for the mental health community but at the same time are aware of its shortcomings, which include:

- Diagnosis labels the individual and may stigmatize them throughout their lives.
- Environmental and social problems are ignored, such as racism and poverty.
- Attention to symptoms and behaviors, not a holistic view.
- Emphasis on medical model treatments, usually medications for symptom relief.
- Racial, cultural, gender bias in diagnosing, for example, over-diagnosing women.

Other negative comments on DSM-IV are that it is nonscientific, has overlapping categories of disorders, and that diagnosis is based on the subjective view of the evaluator, most of whom are white, male psychiatrists. Also, that the symptoms and behaviors diagnosed as a particular disorder may have any number of causes and call for different treatments than are usually prescribed.

CHAPTER 2

Mind and Body

When you are confronted with a stressor, both the mind and body react, resulting in anxiety symptoms. You respond with a survival reaction, called the fight or flight response, which initiates acute changes in every organ, muscle, and limb. Basically, it is the nervous system's response to stressors that triggers anxiety. Anxiety is a natural human quality, but your body and mind can also over-react. The question is: how can you tell that anxiety has ceased to be a normal human reaction and become a chronic problem?

Responding to Stress

Life is full of stress. Daily annoyances, like being stuck in a traffic jam, or more nerve-racking events, like getting married or having a baby, all have to be dealt with in some way. Humans are built to handle stress with primordial defense mechanisms; these help the body make physical and emotional adjustments to meet these situations. When the event or circumstance is over, the body returns to a relaxed state.

In 1925, Hans Selye, a European physician recognized two kinds of stress. The first, eustress, is positive and occurs when buying a new house, competing in the Olympics, or falling in love. These stressors may inspire anxious symptoms, such as sweaty palms when you sign for a new mortgage, an adrenaline rush when the race starts, or increased heart rate when you see your beloved. These events are desired and pleasurable, contributing to a person's sense of achievement and well-being, making the symptoms benign and manageable.

Alert

The words "anxiety" and "stress" are used synonymously, but there can be differences in their meanings. Stress is defined as physical or emotional strain, tension, and pressure, usually in response to known situations that overtax you. On the other hand, anxiety is feelings and emotions that may have no tangible stimulus.

Distress, the second type of stress, is disturbing and harmful and causes discomfort and psychic pain. Being fired, enduring a disabling injury, or getting a DUI summons may cause the same symptoms experienced in positively stressful situations. However, the sweaty palms, adrenaline rush, and rapid heartbeat are now negative and upsetting.

Comparing Anxiety and Stress

Stress can manifest itself in many ways; it can feel like frustration, pressure, exhaustion, or even fear. And how you handle daily stress and cumulative stress over time may be a factor in the development of an anxiety disorder. But it is the seemingly unfounded discomfort, apprehension, and persistence of chronic anxiety that set it apart from basic stress.

How people manage positive and negative stress is determined by many factors, including heredity, childhood experiences, health, and the number of stressors hitting at once. Seyle's contention is that it does not matter whether you are facing something pleasant or unpleasant, what is important is your ability to adapt—to make adjustments to accommodate life's ups and downs.

The Social Readjustment Scale

In 1967, Drs. Richard Thomas and Thomas Rahe devised the Social Readjustment Scale, also known as the Life Events Survey, to predict the likelihood of an individual getting physically ill or having mental health problems when faced with major life changes that occurred within one year. A sampling of the forty-three listed life events include:

- Death of a spouse
- Divorce
- Major personal injury or illness
- Marriage
- Retirement
- Pregnancy
- Major change in financial status
- Change to a new school
- Vacation
- Minor violations of the law (e.g., traffic tickets)

Fact

A recent example of adaptation is Bethany Hamilton, the thirteen-year-old surfer, who dreamed of being a world champion, but lost her arm to a shark in 2003. Within months of the attack she was surfing and competing again. When interviewed after the attack, Bethany said of her situation, that everything was more challenging, but it hadn't changed her personality or outlook on life.

Each event is scored and ranked in order of severity; for example, death of a spouse scores 100 and minor violation of the law scores eleven. The scores are then added, and if your total score is 150 or above it can be assumed you are probably suffering from chronic stress. See the complete survey online by putting "Life Events Survey" into your search engine.

As Seyle maintains, it is your perception of the situation or event and how you react to it that determines its effect upon you. And whether the stressor is small or big, good or bad, the biological process that produces the adrenaline rush and other bodily changes is the same—the fight or flight reaction.

Alert

> If you have recently had a number of changes in your life, you need to recognize how you feel both physically and mentally. For example, take note if you have experienced changes in sleeping or eating patterns or in other daily functioning. Once you know the score, you can take action.

The Nervous System

To know why and how fight or flight affects you, you have to understand its complex processes. It all begins in the nervous system, an intricate group of nerves and organs, which is the body's central organizer, controlling all life functions, breathing, thinking, emotions, reactions, movement of limbs, and organ activity. Nerves are made up of groups of nerve cells, or neurons, that carry messages, called impulses, to every part of the body. There are three types of neurons:

- *Sensory nerve cells*: respond to stimuli in the environment and pass this information on to the brain and spinal cord
- *Motor nerve cells*: carry messages from the brain and spinal cord to muscles and glands
- *Connecting nerve cells*: link sensory and motor nerve cells in the brain and spinal cord

The main function of this communication system is to collect information about conditions in the external environment, inform the body what is going on, and prepare a suitable response, if necessary.

Remember Joe from Chapter 1 who had to swerve his car to avoid an accident? When the oncoming car veered toward his, his nervous system went into action. Sensory cells in Joe's eyes sent impulses to his brain. The brain interpreted that this was a dangerous situation and sent impulses to the muscles in Joe's arms and hands, and he swerved to avoid being hit. All of this happened in a split second. Joe didn't have to think about what he should do, he acted instinctively and relied on his nervous system for survival.

The nervous system is divided into two parts: the central nervous system, which houses the spinal cord and brain; and the peripheral nervous system, which lies outside of the brain and spinal cord. The peripheral nervous system has two divisions. One is the somatic nervous system, which sends sensory information about the external environment to the brain and spinal cord. The other, the autonomic nervous system, controls involuntary functions, like heartbeat and breathing, and is affected by emotions. The autonomic nervous system is divided into the sympathetic and parasympathetic nervous systems.

Essential

It is important to learn about the parts of the brain to understand what happens when the fight or flight response kicks in and panic follows. Sometimes, just knowing where the symptoms come from helps to ease the anxiety. For example, if you know that an adrenaline rush causes heart palpitations, you might be less likely to think that you are dying.

The Central Nervous System

The central nervous system has two divisions: the spinal cord, located in the vertebral cavity, and the brain, located in the brain cavity. The brain is enclosed within the skull and protected by fluid, which acts as a shock absorber. The central nervous system controls mental activity, and muscle and organ functioning. Its 100 billion plus neurons transmit and receive information to and from all parts of the body.

The Brain

The human brain has evolved over millions of years and is the most complex organ known to man. Even to this day, scientists are still attempting to uncover all of its mysteries. This approximately two pound mass of gray matter, containing billions of nerve cells and located in the protective cranium, is responsible for controlling every organ and bodily function.

Chemicals of the Brain

The brain manufactures chemicals, or hormones, called neurotransmitters that affect your physical health and influence moods and thought. Sixty neurotransmitters have been identified. Listed below are five that are commonly known and important in learning about anxiety:

- *Dopamine*: regulates physical movement and emotion
- *Serotonin*: affects mood and anxiety
- *Acetylcholine (Ach)*: controls attention, memory, and learning
- *Noradrenaline*: produces physical and mental arousal and elevated mood
- *Glutamate*: forms links between neurons that control learning and long-term memory
- *Endorphins*: ease pain, reduce stress, and promote tranquility

Research indicates that neurotransmitters can be affected by what we do or think. For example, serotonin levels that affect anxiety may decrease because of chronic stress or increase due to feelings of happiness and a healthy lifestyle. These studies tell us that we are able to take charge of our emotions, and that anxiety does not have to rule our lives.

Parts of the Brain

The brain consists of three main parts:

- *Brain stem (reptilian brain)*: the medulla oblongata controls unconscious, automatic functions such as breathing, heartbeat, and blood pressure. Its cerebellum controls and regulates muscles, movement, and balance.
- *Midbrain*: the thalamus relays information. The hypothalamus regulates drives and actions and is part of the limbic system, which is the center of emotions and drives.

- *Cerebrum*: the largest and newest part of the brain on the evo-lutionary scale. It controls higher functions, such as thought, logic, language, voluntary muscle movement, decision making, and perception.

By studying the brain and its functions, it is understandable why the symptoms of anxiety shake up your system and make a powerful impact on your mind and body, from physiological processes, such as rapid heart rate, and trembling hands, to the inability to concentrate and memory loss.

The Spinal Cord

The spinal cord, a thin column of nerves, comprised of both sensory and motor neurons, is the main highway for sending and receiving information between the central nervous system (brain and spine), and the peripheral nervous system (sensory and motor neurons). The spinal column, which protects the spinal cord, is comprised of twenty-four small bones, with a gel-like disc between each vertebra that act as shock absorbers, and keep bones from rubbing against each other. Not only does the spinal cord allow you to control body movements, but without it, organs would not be able to function. When people have spinal cord injuries, depending on the severity of the injury and which vertebrae were damaged, they may not be able to walk and sometimes will require a respirator to breathe.

The Peripheral Nervous System

The peripheral nervous system consists of cranial nerves that control the structures of the head, and spinal nerves that control all other body functions. It is one of two components of the central nervous system and has two parts: the somatic nervous system and the autonomic nervous system.

The somatic nervous system is an information relaying structure. Twelve pairs of cranial nerves and thirty-one pairs of spinal nerves, contained in blood, lymph glands, internal and sense organs, and muscles, tendons and skin, carry sensory information to the brain and spinal cord. The somatic nervous system tells the brain what is happening both internally and externally, so it can prepare a suitable response.

Fact

The twelve cranial nerves control various important functions of the human body. These functions include both sensory and motor roles. Sensory functions are smell, vision, taste, hearing, and touch. The motor functions include chewing, eye movement, balance, and facial expression.

The autonomic nervous system, made up mostly of motor neurons, is responsible for controlling involuntary responses by sending out hormones and electrical impulses to the heart, lungs, stomach, intestines, liver, kidneys, sweat glands, salivary glands, and pupils of the eyes. It can slow down or speed up the body's organs and systems depending on the situation. The fight or flight reaction will be triggered if danger arises, and when the threat passes, the body will return to its normal resting state. The interaction of its two complimentary branches, the sympathetic nervous system, and the parasympathetic nervous system, keep the body balanced and working properly. But chronic stress can disturb this harmony, leading to anxiety related health problems.

The sympathetic nervous system readies the body to meet threatening or dangerous situations by revving up its defenses to meet the threat, and activating the fight or flight response. The parasympathetic nervous system activates the relaxation response when the all clear is sounded, renewing the body's resources while waiting for the next threat.

Fight or Flight

The fight or flight response, which is triggered when anxiety hits, is a powerful reaction and bears detailing. It is important to understand this process to be able to deal with it better. Whether a real threat occurs (you encounter an angry grizzly bear while hiking), or you simply perceive a threat (you're worried about an upcoming meeting with your boss), your brain recognizes or interprets danger and mobilizes the fight or flight.

Essential

The brain is an amazing organ, but it cannot distinguish the difference between real or perceived danger. The brain mobilizes its defenses to meet both real and perceived danger, setting off acute bodily changes in preparation to fight or to flee.

Without any conscious thought your body responds to danger with certain changes, which take place instantly. The number and intensity of the changes depends on the severity of the threat. Heart rate and blood pressure increase to pump more blood into the brain and muscles, necessary to take swift action. Breathing becomes rapid and deeper to ensure that you get enough oxygen. There is an increase in muscle tension, and adrenaline and other stress hormones are released into the bloodstream. Pupils dilate for more light, and a better view of the threat. A cold sweat may occur to prepare your body for the heat of battle. A decreased production of saliva suspends digestion. Voiding of bowel and bladder makes the body ready for arduous activity.

If you meet up with that grizzly bear in the woods, you might try to run away, you might curl up on the ground and play dead, or you might even try to scare the bear away. No matter what action you take, you will expend a lot of energy defending your life. However, in the meeting with your boss, all of the bodily preparations for battle or retreat have no outlet. Without physical exertion, there is no release. And since you probably can't avoid the meeting, no matter how nervous you are, the brain keeps getting the message that there is danger. The fight or flight symptoms do not abate, you stay tense, and there is a good chance you feel trapped and helpless when you are speaking. Symptoms like these can indicate chronic anxiety and can take over your life if not dealt with promptly.

The Relaxation Response

Once the sympathetic nervous system has done its job to protect you, what happens next? Under normal circumstances, the parasympathetic nervous system activates to return the body back to a non-stressed resting state. Adrenaline and other stress hormones decrease, breathing and blood pressure return to normal, and the digestive system starts functioning. Your muscles relax and you once again feel calm. This primordial process of balance or homeostasis ensures your survival. The resting state is a time of renewing resources, so that when danger strikes again, your defenses will be ready.

Essential

A whole industry has sprung up to help people with anxiety. Go to any bookstore and you'll see shelves filled with self-help books on beating stress. You can find classes for stress management, yoga, meditation, breath-work, and the like. Mental health practitioners offer various techniques to ease anxiety and relax in stressful situations, such as hypnotherapy.

Since the modern world is stressful a good part of the time, it is very difficult to turn off the anxious sympathetic response and turn on the parasympathetic resting state. Most people's lives offer little chance to really relax and renew—two vacation weeks a year can't erase fifty anxious weeks of responsibility and tension. Those with chronic anxiety have to work on creating the relaxation response. Luckily, there are remedies to help you relax, from aromatherapy to Bach flower remedies, special diets, vitamins, herbs, and massage. Whatever the means, learning how to relax and de-stress will benefit your mental and physical health, and lead to a richer contented life.

When Anxiety Becomes Chronic

The fight or flight response is a defense mechanism that is meant for survival of the species. It is a short-term response to a dangerous situation, and as soon as the danger retreats, the body should return to normal and renew itself. But if you continuously suffer anxiety and never go into the relaxation state, the condition may become chronic and you may be susceptible to illness.

Fact

The fight or flight reaction is the defense mechanism for survival of the species, and all animals have the same response to danger. But it is meant to be a short-term response to a present physical threat, not an ongoing state as it often is for many people in today's fast-paced society. Continuing anxiety symptoms left unrelieved can cause serious harm.

When the stress response becomes chronic, it can negatively affect physical health. As mentioned before, when you are frightened your brain sends messages through the spinal cord to parts of the body to prepare to defend itself by releasing stress hormones, such as adrenaline and cortisol, that trigger other physical responses. Some parts of the body turn off, while others go into overdrive to provide the necessary resources needed to survive. It is these acute changes that disrupt the body's balance and functioning and can lead to damaging effects over time on both physical and mental health. Chronic anxiety may lead to:

- Depressed immune system
- Cardiovascular disease
- Cancer
- Stroke
- High blood pressure
- Depression and other mental conditions

There is no magic cure for chronic anxiety. Tranquilizers and other medications can ease symptoms but are not truly cures. Medications have side effects and do not change patterns of thinking and behavior. It seems that the best way to handle chronic stress is a multidimensional approach that involves major lifestyle changes, like learning how to manage stress positively, and giving up smoking and junk food.

General Symptoms of Anxiety

The symptoms of anxiety can be disturbing and even terrifying, but these are just sensations and there is a physiological explanation for them. The following list includes the most common symptoms reported and why they occur. As mentioned earlier, anxiety is an experience unique to each person, so you or someone you know may experience symptoms not listed here.

Physical Symptoms

The physical symptoms of anxiety involve physiological responses, muscle tension, and change in motor function, which also impacts your mental functioning. If you feel physically stiff, awkward, and unbalanced, you will most likely feel mentally unstable as well. The physical symptoms of anxiety are as follows:

- *Rapid heartbeat, palpitations, and slow heart beat*: Any of these might happen when stress hormones, such as adrenaline are released into the bloodstream.
- *Shortness of breath or feelings of being smothered*: When fight or flight kicks in, breathing becomes rapid and shallow and can lead to hyperventilation. Acute fear and feelings of being trapped may lead to the sensation of being smothered.
- *Chest pain*: Caused by extreme muscle tension and leads to fears of having a heart attack.
- *Inability to swallow, or feeling of a lump in the throat*: Caused by contractions of throat muscles due to tension.

- *Shaking, trembling, and shivering*: When we get afraid body temperature drops and we shake to warm ourselves.
- *Sweating*: Occurs when the body cools to prepare for arduous activity.
- *Tingling and numbness*: Changes in hormones and more blood pumped into muscles will create any of these sensations.
- *Numbness in head and face*: Muscles in face become tense due to increased stress.
- *Blanching*: When you are frightened, you lose skin color because blood is diverted to muscles needed for battle, so blood vessels in your face constrict.
- *Diarrhea/constipation/frequent voiding*: Blood is diverted away from stomach to other areas, digestion slows, and muscles tighten leading to stomach problems.

Some people suffering from anxiety may also experience skin problems, as anxiety disturbs nerve endings in the skin, causing numbness and itchy sensations. Dry mouth often occurs because body fluids are sent to other areas, making the mouth uncomfortably dry. Your pupils may dilate and become hypersensitive to light or you may experience distorted vision, such as tunnel vision. Headaches can also occur because the blood vessels in the head constrict causing pain in the face, head, shoulders, and neck. Anxiety may even affect your hearing. Additionally, adrenaline increases the amount of sugar in the bloodstream and raises the heart rate. Cortisol keeps blood sugar high, and blood pressure up, making sure the body has the energy to defend itself. Studies have found that long-term elevated levels of cortisol are harmful to both physical and mental functioning.

Mental and Emotional Symptoms

The mental and emotional symptoms of anxiety affect all cognitive functions. When you get anxious you may find it hard to think clearly and to handle your emotions. There's a fear that you will lose control of yourself, and wonder how you will continue to live this way. Some of the symptoms are mild, but many can be frightening and debilitating. Some mental and emotional symptoms of anxiety are as follows:

- *Anger/aggression*: Anxiety can lead you to feel frustrated and irritable. Some of this tension might release itself in the form of anger or aggression.
- *Feeling jittery*: Some anxiety sufferers find it hard to sit still and concentrate on tasks at hand.
- *Feeling shocks*: Anxiety can cause abnormal nerve impulses that result in many strange sensations, like the feeling of being jolted with electricity.
- *Suicidal thoughts*: When anxiety becomes severe, with seemingly no way to stop it, feelings of hopelessness and despair are common.
- *Fear of losing control/going crazy*: Changes in blood flow, hormones, muscle tension, nerves, etc., exhaust the mind, creating distorted thinking.

Other emotional and mental symptoms you may experience include: avoidance (straying from things that frighten you), depression, and sleep difficulties (such as insomnia and nightmares). Hyperfocusing on the anxiety and ceasing to do the things that make life enjoyable are also common responses. Anxiety sufferers may feel shame because they see themselves as weak. Feelings of "depersonalization," feeling out of one's body, self-hatred, hopelessness, and low self-worth are also prevalent in people with anxiety disorders.

Anxiety is a complex condition that affects your overall mental and physical well-being. Now that you know a bit more about how the brain works, and what happens when it reacts to danger, whether real or imagined, you can see why an anxiety disorder can make daily living so challenging.

CHAPTER 3

Panic Disorder

One of the many intricacies in the world of anxiety is panic disorder. Those suffering from panic disorder experience unique symptoms, the most recognizable of which is the panic attack. There are different kinds of panic disorders, each with its own characteristic symptoms and treatments. To know if you have a panic disorder, it's important to learn about the possibilities. This chapter will discuss the differences between the disorders, their symptoms, causes, criteria for diagnosis, and treatments.

Panic Attacks

A panic attack is a sudden wave of paralyzing fear that begins without warning for no apparent reason and seems to have no solution. The feelings are so acute and terrifying that people who experience them may feel like they are out of control, losing their minds, or dying, and they usually flee the situation. Panic attacks are not considered a stand-alone disorder according to the DSM-IV, but they are an aspect of a number of mental disorders.

The symptoms used for diagnosis of panic attacks include: pounding heart or palpitations, shortness of breath or feeling smothered, feeling shaky or trembling, sweating, choking sensations, chest pain, dizziness or lightheadedness, fear that one is going crazy, feeling unsteady or faint, nausea and abdominal distress, numbness, feeling cold or hot, distorted perception of the external world, and fear of dying. To be formally diagnosed as having had a panic attack, you must experience at least four of the above symptoms. If only two or three are present it is referred to as a limited-symptom attack.

Essential

Many panic attack sufferers wind up in hospital emergency rooms during or after attacks. In fact, it is estimated that individuals with panic attacks visit doctors ten times more often than people without panic, and they go to emergency rooms fifteen times more than people who don't have panic attacks.

Features of Panic Attacks

If you experience a panic attack, you may not perceive any threat or danger. Panic attacks peak in approximately ten minutes but can last as long as thirty minutes. Some people report their panic peaking and subsiding for hours. Repeated attacks usually vary in intensity and sometimes never reach the severity of the first attack.

Panic attacks may come on suddenly without warning and may not be brought on by any particular stimulus. These are referred to as spontaneous (uncued) panic attacks and can strike when you are in relaxed situations—while at home watching TV or sleeping, for example. Situational (cued) panic attacks occur when you either anticipate having panic or have had an attack in feared situations; for example, being socially phobic or having performance anxiety. Situational predisposed panic attacks happen when you are susceptible to panic in a situation. For example, you may sometimes have attacks in restaurants, and other times not.

Whatever kind of panic attacks you experience, and whatever your level of discomfort, the symptoms are not dangerous. They are only feelings and sensations and cannot hurt you. The unpredictability of panic, the feelings of being completely out of control, and not knowing what is wrong with you are what makes these panic attacks so difficult to cope with.

Free-Floating Anxiety

Free-floating anxiety is severe and persistent and cannot be attributed to a particular situation, event, or object. For instance, if you are sitting on the couch watching TV and you suddenly get panicky, this could be free-floating anxiety. It is often found in people with panic disorder. Free-floating anxiety is frightening because you never know when it will hit. You might subconsciously connect your feelings with situations or places where the panic happened, but it is not those events or places that make you so frightened. The distinctive signature of panic attacks is the fear of the fear. Marge's experience is a typical example:

> While doing her usual weekly supermarket shopping, as Marge reaches for a jar of peanut butter, she has her first panic attack. Heart pounding, sweating, and chest pains lead Marge to believe she was having a heart attack. Leaving the store, she drives herself to the hospital emergency room, and after a number of tests, she is diagnosed with anxiety, given a tranquilizer, and sent home. But Marge's intense physical symptoms were exactly those of a heart attack, and she does not believe it was anxiety induced. Marge continues to go on thinking she's having a heart attack when the panic begins. And another attack does occur in the same supermarket. Then the attacks spread to other stores, when she's driving, while she's at work, and even when she's home alone. She continues to function in her daily life, going to stores, driving, etc., but does so under great stress, waiting for a heart attack. Eventually, she becomes obsessed with taking her pulse as soon as she feels anxiety starting. And even after seeing many doctors, and taking every possible test for cardiovascular disease, all with negative results, she has begun carrying a map in her car outlined with the shortest routes to the area hospitals.

Panic Linked to Illness

The real fear in panic disorder is fear of another attack. And though the symptoms and sensations are not dangerous, panic disorder is no laughing matter. If you do not seek treatment, panic disorder can become as disabling to your life and physical and mental health as any serious physical injury or disease.

Panic disorder can take time to diagnose, or lead to misdiagnosis if your family physician is not well informed about anxiety disorders. This is because the symptoms associated with it mirror any number of medical conditions, including the following:

- Heart arrhythmia
- Mitral valve prolapse
- Colitis
- Hyperthyroidism
- Hypoglycemia
- Hypertension

If you have had repeated panic attacks, and seek medical attention, it is important for the doctor to do extensive testing to rule out the possibility of a medical condition. Maybe you believe you have a physical illness and have gone to many doctors trying to find relief. But the most important step after ruling out a medical condition is a referral to a mental health professional specializing in the diagnosis and treatment of anxiety disorders. Some people have repeated attacks, sometimes on a daily basis, and do develop a panic disorder. However, though they may report some avoidance, they mostly continue doing what they have to do to fulfill their responsibilities in life.

Agoraphobia

As more attacks occur, a state of "anticipatory anxiety," a state of apprehension caused by waiting for the next attack, is created. This increases both physical and mental stress and strain. Agoraphobia is the fear of having panic attacks or the feelings of panic and of being trapped in situations or places where there seems to be no way to escape.

People diagnosed with panic disorder may not develop agoraphobia, but according to the National Institute of Mental Health (NIMH), approximately one-third of people with panic disorder become agoraphobic, and other studies show that this occurs within a year of the initial panic attack. Agoraphobia may develop after the first attack, or a year or more later, but as with all anxiety, it is a different experience for everyone. There are instances in the medical literature of cases with twenty or more years between attacks, or people having one attack but never having another one ever again. Take a look at Helen's case:

Helen is twenty-eight years old, married, and a stay at home mom with two children in elementary school. One day after Helen sees the kids off to school, she decides to go to the mall—a place she's been to hundreds of times. While she is standing in line waiting to check out, she begins to feel nervous and within seconds is hit with a panic attack. The ferocity of the sensations is terrifying. She trembles, can barely catch her breath, and feels like she's suffocating. She feels dizzy and stumbles out of line. Her surroundings take on a dreamlike quality, and all movement around her is in slow motion.

What frightens Helen the most is how detached from herself she feels. (She later describes it as an out-of-body experience.) She feels helpless and unprotected. When she notices people staring at her, she drops the clothes she is holding and begins frantically looking for an exit. Her one thought is to get home where she will be safe, and as she drives home thinking about what occurred, she is sure that she is going crazy. On the way home the panic subsides, but the fear about what happened is still palpable.

Her husband tries to reassure her that she is not going crazy, but she remains obsessed about her sanity. After a long, disturbing night, Helen is still shaky the next day, but in the morning, she goes to the supermarket. On the way there she begins thinking about yesterday at the mall and is suddenly hit with another attack. Frantic, she drives home and calls her husband at work to come home. As the attacks continue over the next months, in cars, stores, in her children's school, movie theaters, and restaurants, Helen begins to avoid these places. She makes excuses to friends and stops going out with them because she is afraid she'll "freak out" and is ashamed to tell them about what's happening to her.

Little by little, her only safety net is being with her husband, and even his presence doesn't help in certain situations. She stops driving alone and only drives short distances. Helen starts putting off family events and visits, and eventually her husband and children have to stop many activities, or her husband goes it alone with their children, explaining to them that "Mommy doesn't feel well." She visits a number of doctors and is extensively tested, but she is misdiagnosed for years. Helen's life soon revolves around doing anything she can to avoid an attack.

Is Helen afraid of cars, the mall, restaurants, and supermarkets? No—she is afraid of the fear, of being trapped, embarrassed, unsafe, and of going crazy. Her world is shrinking. She could well become housebound if she does not get properly diagnosed and correctly treated.

Fact

Agorphobia comes from the Greek words, "agora," meaning marketplace, and "phobia," meaning fear ("fear of the marketplace"). The term was coined by psychiatrist Karl Friedrich Westphal in 1871 in his study of men who had panic attacks in public places. Agoraphobia has been referred to as the "fear of open spaces" in the past, but that definition has since broadened.

Once individuals move toward avoidance, the effects of agoraphobia spread over every part of their lives. Since one of the nastier features of panic attacks is its element of surprise, it's no wonder that people would prefer a coping style of staying in a safe place, than going out and facing the very real possibility of another attack.

Common places and situations that agoraphobics avoid have characteristics that lend themselves to feeling trapped and vulnerable. Some of these places include public transportation like airplanes, buses, and trains. And many people avoid situations in which they are home alone or driving alone, and they also avoid being far from home. Like Helen, many people with agoraphobia find a "safe person," either a trusted family member or friend to rely on in fearful situations. Some people carry bottles of water in case they feel choking sensations and medications in case of an attack.

L. Essential

It is estimated that 10 percent of people who develop agoraphobia will become housebound, unable to leave home alone. To show how serious panic disorder can become, cases in agoraphobia literature include people who wouldn't even venture out to get their mail, and some who locked themselves in their homes for decades.

Different Panic Disorders

All panic disorders have major similarities in symptoms and behaviors. The differences may seem slight, but they're very important. The presence or absence of panic attacks or agoraphobia in a person's condition may warrant a particular course of treatment.

Panic Disorder Without Agoraphobia

The main characteristic of panic disorder without agoraphobia is recurrent panic attacks that are out of proportion to the situation at hand, coupled with anticipatory worry about getting future attacks, losing control, dying, and so on. Most people with panic disorder eventually exhibit some avoidance behavior, but they may not necessarily develop agoraphobia. It is this difference that defines the diagnosis, for it cannot include the more serious agoraphobic behaviors. Other criteria for diagnosis are the absence of substance abuse or having another anxiety disorder.

Panic Disorder with Agoraphobia

The essential elements of this diagnosis are persistent panic attacks, and at least one of the attacks has to be followed by one or more months of at least one of the following:

- Great distress that other attacks will follow
- Apprehension about what the attacks mean
- Critical changes in behavior after attacks

Of course, also included is the eventual development of agoraphobia, which will lead to avoidance behavior and severe restrictions on the ability to function in daily life. Research shows that about 90 percent of people who report having agoraphobia, experience panic attacks.

Agoraphobia Without History of Panic Disorder

There a few fundamental elements of agoraphobia without panic disorder. The focal point of the anxiety is fear of having symptoms of panic in a place or circumstance where there is no help and escape will be difficult and embarrassing. Also, those who experience symptoms of agoraphobia, such as dizziness, but do not have panic attacks, or have only limited-symptom attacks, are probably suffering from this condition.

It is estimated that 10 percent of people diagnosed have agoraphobia without having full-blown panic attacks, but studies show that the longer agoraphobia is present, the more likely it is that panic attacks will develop.

One reason why agoraphobia may develop without panic attacks is that people start avoiding as soon as they begin experiencing anxiety, thus never allowing themselves to be in situations that might cause an attack. Agoraphobia also appears in other disorders besides panic disorder, such as obsessive-compulsive disorder (one of the anxiety disorders) and in the bipolar disorders (classified under mood disorders).

Fact

Bipolar disorder is characterized by swings of depressive periods alternating with manic occurrences and offset by extended periods of relatively normal behavior. Among associated mental disorders, DSM-IV includes panic disorders and social phobias.

Variations in Panic Symptoms and Effects

Though each diagnosis has its specifics, panic disorders share common features besides the physiology of panic attacks. Panic attacks vary in recurrence and intensity; you may have attacks daily or weekly, for months at a time, and then experience weeks or months without attacks. Some people have periods of intense attacks, then become symptom-free for years, with panic suddenly returning after decades. You may have a few panic attacks per month every year, or one or two attacks in a year. These attacks can range from full-blown to limited and be spontaneous or situational.

L. Essential

It is estimated that approximately 40 percent of people with panic disorder suffer from depression. Since depression carries some of the same symptoms as anxiety disorders, such as stress, insomnia, and difficulty concentrating, proper diagnosis is difficult. Therefore, it is important to be evaluated for depression too, to be sure your anxiety treatment is appropriate.

No matter how panic disorder manifests itself, a number of problems may arise that create additional stress and strain emotionally, personally, and professionally. The effect of panic disorder on interpersonal relationships is enormous, sometimes leading to family crises and divorce. Professional and educational situations are compromised due to absenteeism, decreased ability to focus, and fear of new situations. Loss of jobs and income, or dropping out of school is common. The inability to handle anxiety increases feelings of being weak, unworthy, and ashamed. Given this information, it makes sense that the majority of people with panic disorder feel hopeless and become disheartened.

Causes of Panic Disorder

The theories that may explain the onset of panic disorder are numerous. However, it is generally believed that a combination of causes exist, including biology, heredity and family patterns, major life stressors, medical conditions, and drug use. Some of these are better understood than others.

Biology

The biology of panic is not completely understood, but it is believed that chemical imbalances between the neurotransmitters in the brain make you more reactive to such external stimuli as light, noise, smells, movement, and medication. For example, you may be hypersensitive to strobe lights, TV screens, bright fluorescents, or sunlight, and these can set off a panic attack. With repeated attacks you may begin to avoid places with similar stimuli, such as nightclubs, movie theaters, and malls. If you have this chemical imbalance, are predisposed to panic attacks, and experience physical and emotional stress, an overload may occur, signaling danger to your body and triggering the flight or fight response.

Heredity and Family Patterns

Research studies conclude that heredity factors may play a part when panic disorders run in families. It is estimated that more than 20 percent of children who have at least one parent with panic disorder will develop it too. Other studies indicate that one half of all people with panic have at least one relative with panic disorder. Whether parenting styles contributed to the results is unknown and more research is needed. Most experts agree that both heredity and learning play an important role in who gets panic disorders and who doesn't.

Family patterns are a combination of heredity and psychological factors. How your parents interact with you and the world directly impacts your personality, feelings of self-worth, and ability to manage life's stressors. People with panic disorder commonly report the following parental characteristics:

- Perpetually tense and anxious
- Suffering from panic and phobias
- Perfectionist
- Overprotective
- Abusive

A number of psychological theories believe unresolved childhood conflict—the issue of breaking away and becoming independent from your parents, for example—may account for a predisposition to panic disorder. Many studies show a connection between parents' fears and anxiety disorder in their children.

Major Life Stressors

Panic may be triggered when you are overwhelmed by a major life event, such as getting divorced, or having to face many stressors all at once, such as getting divorced and having to move and look for a job, all while a parent is seriously ill. Other negative life stressors include death of a loved one, having a chronic disease, facing a natural disaster, and losing your job. Even "happy" events may initiate panic, such as moving away from home to go to college, getting married, and becoming a parent. All these events create distress until you acclimate to the change.

Fact

Studies have shown that new mothers are at risk for panic disorders, but only during the first four months after birth. As they become accustomed to the role of motherhood, the panic usually stops. Some of these mothers might also be at risk for postpartum depression.

Medical Conditions

A number of medical conditions account for panic attacks, but if panic does occur for these reasons, it does not necessarily mean that you will develop a panic disorder. The symptoms produced by illnesses or other conditions mirror those of panic disorders, so a thorough physical exam is important to determine if you have a medical condition and determine what treatment you need. Some of these medical conditions include:

- *Pulmonary disease*: Decreases levels of oxygen, leading to feelings of anxiety.
- *Mitral valve prolapse*: Causes heart palpitations.
- *Chronic hyperventilation*: Creates shortness of breath, and heart palpitations.
- *Hypoglycemia*: Leads to heart palpitations, sweating, and anxiety.
- *Meniere's syndrome/inner ear disturbances*: Cause feelings of being lightheaded and dizzy.
- *Hyperthyroidism*: Imbalance in thyroid results in high blood pressure and rapid heartbeat.

If panic disorder does not exist as a separate condition once these problems are treated, then the symptoms should disappear.

Fact

About 30 percent of people with panic use alcohol, 17 percent abuse drugs such as marijuana and cocaine, more than society's norm smoke, and an unknown percentage continue to use methamphetamine and the current designer drugs, all putting themselves at risk for anxiety leading to panic disorders.

Drug Use

Over-the-counter medications, prescription medications, and legal and illegal recreational drugs can cause symptoms associated with panic attacks. It is important for you to provide your drug history to your doctor for proper diagnosis. The drugs commonly associated with panic attacks are blood pressure medications, steroids, thyroid medications, cold and allergy drugs, tranquilizers, and sleeping pills.

Substances such as caffeine, nicotine, and alcohol can cause trembling, shaking, and dizziness. Drugs like marijuana can lead to anxious feelings. Stimulants, such as cocaine, and methamphetamines create a "rush," and in long-term use can lead to anxiety. Hallucinogens, such as LSD and Ecstasy, can cause dizziness and lead to panic and psychotic reactions. Withdrawal of some of the above can also create anxious symptoms.

Age Considerations

For unknown reasons, panic disorders most frequently appear between the ages of fifteen and twenty-five. Though rare, children report the same panic symptoms that adults do, with stomach aches and headaches being common. Both children and adults are likely to have more than one anxiety disorder, and anxiety sufferers are also known to experience depression and phobias. With little research done on the aging population, experts of the past thought that older adults outgrew or did not develop anxiety disorders.

Essential

At one time it was believed that younger children and adults over fifty did not develop panic disorders. However, current information and research indicates that both these populations do suffer from panic disorder. Young children may experience panic attacks with separation-anxiety disorder, and older adults can have panic disorders and agoraphobia.

Research has shown that many older adults experienced an anxiety disorder earlier in their lives and might have been in remission of symptoms for many years. As they aged, major life events and changes, such as significant losses, like death of a spouse, physical illness, and deteriorating cognitive abilities, and other mental disorders such as major depression, placed them at a high risk for developing anxiety disorders. It is paramount that this population be properly diagnosed to receive correct care and treatment.

Distinctions Between Genders and Cultures

It is believed that women are twice as likely to develop panic disorder without agoraphobia than men and are three times as likely to have panic disorder with agoraphobia. Studies and researchers have proposed a number of explanations for these differences, which include:

- "Nervous problems" are associated more with women than men.
- Women ask for help more than men, who do not want to seem "weak."
- Men have a higher rate than women of self-medicating with alcohol and drugs.

Studies indicate that men are more resistant than women to admitting they have an anxiety disorder, because cultural beliefs state that emotional problems are female oriented. Other factors include: social pressures on women (such as multiple roles and multitasking), domestic and sexual violence, and an increase in women's substance abuse.

Cross-cultural studies in the prevalence of panic disorders indicate that it is found worldwide. Many cultures see little value in mental health services, and diagnosing and treating panic in other cultures from a Western perspective is difficult because of cultural differences. The differences include cultural views about the causes of mental distress, attitudes about women, stigma and shame in seeking treatment, racism and ignorance regarding cultural differences in the Western mental health community, poverty, and inaccessibility of health care.

Fact

Studies show that minorities are at a high risk for anxiety and depression due to racism and discrimination, and that people living in poverty are two to three times more likely to have a mental disorder than those in the top socioeconomic group who have access to health care.

Diagnosis

As previously mentioned, diagnosing panic disorder is difficult, as many conditions mimic panic symptoms, and other variables, such as gender and culture, can make a condition difficult to identify. The typical scenario may begin with a person going to the hospital emergency room after the first attack, and possibly being told that they've had an anxiety attack. The next step will be a visit to the primary care physician for a complete physical exam and testing.

Mental health experts base their diagnosis on the reported symptoms and their intensity, the frequency of the attacks, the patient's behavior and mood, and the patient's history and family history. The DSM-IV is used as a guide by listing criteria and diagnostic features. Psychiatrists and other mental health professionals may also utilize interviews and special assessment tools to determine the diagnosis for panic disorder.

Question

What will a family physician look for in a person who has supposedly had an anxiety attack?
The family physician will check for symptoms of a heart condition and any illnesses, such as hyperthyroidism. Testing will most likely include blood screening, EKG, thyroid test, etc. If the family physician suspects an anxiety disorder, then a referral to a mental health professional is made.

If you have panic disorder you may have other emotional conditions as well. Research shows that between 50 percent and 65 percent of people with panic have major depressive disorder or another anxiety disorder. Abusing drugs or alcohol as a way to cope with anxiety is common. Irritable bowel syndrome is also often linked to stress and anxiety. Other mental conditions associated with anxiety disorders are suicide attempts, migraines, and chronic pain. Experts and researchers continue to study the connection between anxiety, physical illnesses, and other mental conditions to be able to make better diagnoses, and to offer sufferers more successful treatments.

Treatment

Just as there are many theories on the causes of panic disorder, there are also differing opinions as to the best course of treatment. The most popular conventional treatments include different types of therapy or counseling, coupled with medication. Cognitive behavioral therapy helps the person to identify thought patterns and behaviors and work on changing them. Psychotherapies consider the emotional causes and help people develop new life strategies. The most prescribed drugs to treat panic disorder are two antidepressants, Paxil and Zoloft, and the anti-anxiety medications, Xanax and Klonopin. Because of medication side-effects, disappointment in the efficacy of conventional treatments, and the mainstreaming of many alternative remedies into Western medicine, many people are turning to alternative therapies to their treatment plan, such as yoga, massage, and acupuncture.

More research is needed into the effectiveness and safety of both conventional and alternative treatments. People with panic disorder are desperately seeking relief from their suffering and a way to lead normal and productive lives. The closest thing to a "cure" for anxiety is usually a multidimensional approach, unique to each individual.

CHAPTER 4

Phobias

The word phobia comes from the Greek, meaning "fear." Phobias are anxiety disorders characterized by excessive fear of things, people, places, and situations, which causes changes in behavior. There are two main types of phobias: specific phobia, which was known in the past as simple phobia, and social phobia, which is also called social anxiety disorder. This chapter elaborates on the differences between specific phobia and social phobia and their symptoms, causes, and treatment possibilities.

Phobia Fundamentals

It is estimated that more than 10 percent of the U.S. population, including children, adolescents, and adults, have phobias. Over 6.3 million Americans have specific phobias, and more than 5.3 million suffer from social phobia. Phobias can occur in conjunction with other anxiety disorders. For example, those with panic disorder may also suffer from agoraphobia, and people with obsessive-compulsive disorder may have hemophobia, the fear of blood.

The phobic response is essentially the "fight or flight" reaction. You see the feared thing, or experience the feared situation; your brain interprets it as dangerous, and your body's defense mechanism is jump-started. There are seemingly countless different phobias, and millions of people suffer from them, including famous people. Napoleon Bonaparte suffered from ailurophobia—fear of cats; Sigmund Freud was an agoraphobe, afraid of unfamiliar places and open spaces; Edgar Allan Poe was claustrophobic, afraid of small spaces; and Aretha Franklin is aerophobic, frightened of flying.

Specific (Simple) Phobia

The basic characteristic of specific phobia is the fear of certain objects or situations that are not usually dangerous or harmful. When you are exposed to the feared stimulus, an anxiety response usually occurs. Depending on your level of fear, and other variables in the situation, your response may range from mild anxiety to a panic attack. For example, if you are afraid of spiders, you may feel a little nervous seeing a picture of one but may have a full-blown panic attack if a spider crawls up your leg. Sometimes the things to which people have phobic reactions are dangerous, such as poisonous snakes, hurricanes, or dark alleys. But if your fear is disproportionate to the situation, it can eventually restrict your life.

L. Essential

Individuals with phobias may also manifest similar symptoms of panic disorder—for example, having frequent panic attacks, and displaying avoidance behavior. The most common symptoms of phobias include rapid heartbeat, sweating, helplessness, avoidance, and feeling lightheaded or faint.

Cued or Predisposed Reaction

The type of panic attack a phobic person will experience may be either a situationally cued panic attack (for example, having a phobic reaction every time you see a cat), or a situationally predisposed panic attack (for instance, having a phobic reaction on a bridge if you are stuck in traffic, but not having a phobic reaction if there is no traffic, and can drive off quickly). If you are phobic there is a good chance you know your fear is extreme and irrational, but are unable to stop your feelings and face your fears.

⬮ Alert

If someone close to you has a phobia, do not force him or her into exposure to the feared thing or situation. For example, do not push someone with hydrophobia into a swimming pool to help them "get over it." The phobic person must be allowed to maintain control of the situation and decide his or her own actions to eventually conquer the fear.

Panic Reactions in Phobias

The anxiety evoked in phobias is often based on specific fears of being harmed by the object or situation, unlike panic disorders, where the anxiety comes "out of the blue." Or the fears may be similar to panic disorders, that is of losing control, being embarrassed, fainting in public, and so on, but that only occurs when anticipating the feared circumstance, or being in it. Examples of panic reactions in phobias include:

- *Fear of dogs*: Afraid of being attacked and bitten.
- *Fear of flying*: Afraid the plane will crash.
- *Fear of small spaces*: Afraid of losing control and screaming.
- *Fear of public speaking*: Afraid you'll forget your speech and feel humiliated.

Many phobias begin in childhood, for example, being afraid of the dark or the fear of animals. These phobias can follow you into adulthood. Children often experience the same physiological reaction to the feared stimulus as adults, with symptoms like crying, freezing, clinging or outbursts, but they are often unaware that their fears are irrational.

Criteria for Diagnosis

As with other anxiety disorders, the symptoms for specific phobia vary according to your unique experience. But to be diagnosed with specific phobia you must meet certain criteria. You have chronic extreme fear that is triggered by being close to or thinking you will come in contact with a specific object or situation. You always have a phobic reaction when you are exposed to your fear. Either you suffer when in contact with the phobic stimulus or avoid it. Your phobic reactions have a major negative impact in your daily life and disrupt your personal and professional life. If you have a child under the age of eighteen, they must have phobic symptoms for at least six months. It must also be established that your symptoms are not due to another anxiety disorder or condition.

However, one of the distinctions in diagnosing specific phobia is the absence of spontaneous panic attacks. In Chapter 3, you learned that phobias may develop alongside panic, as in agoraphobia. But agoraphobia will not develop into specific phobia, because the person with specific phobia is not afraid of having a panic attack. There is no "fear of the fear"—it is the phobic stimulus, such as a spider, that frightens.

Types of Specific Phobias

Specific phobias are divided into subtypes. It is possible to suffer from more than one thing within a subtype; for example, fearing both dogs and spiders. And one can have phobias from different subtypes, such as, being afraid of frogs and public transportation. The subtypes for specific phobias are:

- *Animal type*: Diagnosed if fear is triggered by animals or insects, such as cats, birds, beetles, and spiders. These phobias usually begin in childhood.
- *Natural environment type*: Diagnosed if the fear is triggered by phenomena found in the natural environment, such as storms, water, earth, and heights. It normally begins in childhood.

- *Blood-injection-injury type*: Diagnosed if the fear is triggered by seeing blood or people injured, or by having an injection, or an invasive medical procedure. This type seems to run in families, and its characteristic symptom is a vasovagal episode, which is a simple faint.

📋 Fact

Vasovagal syncope or simple faint occurs when the autonomic nervous system is overloaded. This response drops blood pressure and causes a slow heart rate. When blood pressure drops, less blood gets to the brain, and fainting occurs.

Situational type is diagnosed if fear is triggered by being in or anticipating a certain situation, such as flying, going over a bridge or through a tunnel, driving, and public speaking. Many people have what is called a "bimodal onset," which means the phobia peaks at two different ages, one in early childhood, the other usually in the mid-twenties. It has similarities to panic disorder with agoraphobia.

Other type is diagnosed if your fear is triggered by phenomena not included in the other subtypes. The fear is sparked by being in situations that might set off symptoms, such as choking, vomiting, or getting sick, for example, being afraid to eat in a restaurant because you might get food poisoning. Other type can begin in childhood, with fears, such as, loud noises.

A major difference between specific phobias and other anxiety disorders, such as social phobia, or generalized anxiety disorder is that specific phobias do not permeate your every waking moment. The phobic reaction only occurs when the feared stimulus is present, or in anticipation of its presence. Though the anxiety may broaden if the feared object cannot be avoided; then panic disorder may develop.

Specific Phobias for Everything

There is a named phobia for pretty much everything in this world. There is even a phobia for being afraid of "everything!" It's true. This phobia is known as panophobia or pantophobia. There are currently more than 500 phobias listed, but as changes occur in the culture, and new technology emerges, someone will become afraid of it, and another name will be added to the list. For example, before the technological age there was no such thing as technophobia.

Animal Phobias

Animal phobias often develop in childhood through learned behavior or an upsetting personal experience. For example, your parent may have had a fear reaction to a spider that scared you, or one dropped onto your head and crawled onto your face. Many of the animals in the phobia list are creatures you have feared since childhood, and as adults still bother you. Here are some examples:

- Dogs—cynophobia
- Snakes—ophidiophobia
- Spiders—arachnophobia
- Bees—apiphobia, melissophobia
- Frogs—batrachophobia

Some animals are considered dangerous, but others simply inspire revulsion or disgust, such as rats, and maggots. However, some people are afraid of animals that most people would find cute or harmless, such as rabbits.

Natural Environment Phobias

Natural environment phobias commonly begin in childhood, most likely due to a frightening experience, or learned from parents' anxious reactions. For example, if a parent fears water, a child may become afraid to learn how to swim. The following list includes some of the more common natural environment phobias.

- Electricity—electrophobia
- Heights—acrophobia
- Hurricanes, tornadoes—lilapsophobia
- Sunshine, daylight—phengophobia
- Water—hydrophobia

Natural environment phobias, like animal phobias may continue into adulthood, and create disruptions and interference in your work and personal situations.

Essential

Phobias are listed for every activity, action, thought process, and object. The fear of walking is ambulophobia, the fear of going to bed is clinophobia, the fear of thinking is phronemophobia, and the fear of clothing is vestiphobia. Names of phobias always seem to be at least ten letters long, and oddly enough, there is even a phobia for long words—hippopotomonstrosesquippedaliophobia.

Blood, Injection, Illness, and Injury Phobias

Blood, injection, illness, and injury phobias differ from other specific phobias because the major symptom is not a panic reaction, but a fainting spell. The fight or flight kicks in initially but is then followed by an immediate change to the resting state that quickly lowers your heart rate and blood pressure. The phobias listed in this type are things that can really hurt or cause worry and fear:

- Injury—traumatophobia
- Injections—trypanophobia
- Blood—hemophobia
- Disease—pathophobia
- Pain—algophobia

Blood, injection, injury, illness phobia often keeps people from having necessary medical procedures. It is differentiated from illness phobia, which is an extreme and irrational fear of having a serious or terminal disease, such as AIDs or cancer. The illness phobia is grouped under the diagnosis hypochondriasis, the preoccupation of having a serious disease based on bodily sensations.

Situational Phobias

The situational phobias are very common in people who are phobic. These phobias can develop in early childhood; for example, at six months old a child can develop a fear of loud noises, or within a year a fear of heights, and later fears of the darkness and being alone. Here are some common situational phobias:

- Being alone—monophobia
- Public speaking—glossophobia
- Fear of darkness—achluophobia
- Flying—aviophobia
- Decisions—deciophobia
- Friday the 13th—paraskavedekatriaphobia

These phobias often persist into adulthood. Aviophobia, the fear of flying, is one of the most common fears of adults, and the fear of public speaking or performing is thought to be the number one fear in the United States. Included in the subtypes is "other type," which includes phobias such as the of fear of expressing opinions, doxophobia; the fear of looking up, anablephobia; and the fear of motion, kinetophobia.

Though many of the phobias seem ridiculous, the person afraid of goldfish has the same distress as the person who is afraid of sharks. Many people with these phobias know that their fear doesn't make sense, but being able to look at the feared stimulus, be near it, or in the feared situation is almost impossible. Trying to do so will set off acute anxiety or a panic attack.

Social Phobia (Social Anxiety Disorder)

Social phobia is characterized by an overwhelming fear of embarrassing yourself in daily social situations. It is a complex disorder and can range from a milder form to a more generalized disorder that can become severe because it pervades every interaction in your personal and professional life. Social phobics are hypersensitive to the feelings and thoughts of being constantly watched and evaluated by others. You may recognize that your feelings and thoughts are irrational but cannot turn off the phobic responses or stop the anxiety. Panic attacks are common and are situational if they occur.

Question

What is arachibutyrophobia?
Arachibutyrophobia is the fear of peanut butter sticking to the roof of one's mouth! Though this fear sounds absurd, people with this phobia can become distressed in the same way that someone with the fear of spiders does. Though seemingly unique, for this phobia to be named, a number of people have had to report the fear as a problem.

Criteria for Diagnosis

If you are diagnosed with social phobia you will experience marked fear, anxiety or panic attacks if you are in a social or performance situation where you will be evaluated. You fear your behavior or actions will humiliate you. For children the interaction must be with peers, and their responses include crying, withdrawing, or tantrums. You may avoid situations, and the anxiety severely disrupts your personal and professional life. Your symptoms can be caused by another mental disorder, such as panic disorder, body dysmorphic disorder, schizoid personality disorder, or pervasive developmental disorder.

When individuals with social phobia seek treatment, they may not volunteer the full range of symptoms they have due to difficulty in facing their problems, shame, and fearing they will be seen as "weak," or "crazy." Social phobia may be difficult to diagnose because it does mimic other disorders such as the panic disorders. It is important for mental health practitioners to ask pertinent questions about social situations to make a correct diagnosis for effective treatment planning.

Living with Social Phobia

The excessive self-consciousness resulting from this disorder can lead to extreme behavior in daily activities, until you are incapable of interaction outside the home. Social phobics have a dread of people who they think are watching them, judging them, and negatively noting the way they eat, drink, speak, walk, or dress. And often accompanying these fears are physical symptoms that may last for years. These include similar symptoms to panic attacks due to the acute nervous response and include sweating, nausea, headaches, twitching, stuttering, blushing, fainting, thought blocking, and even temporary hearing loss has been reported.

The variety of social situations and symptoms associated with social phobia is vast. Some of the more common behaviors and circumstances that make functioning with social phobia so difficult either make you feel like you are in the spotlight, or that your anxiety will be noticed. These include:

- Being the center of attention.
- Being watched while engaged in activities, such as eating.
- Meeting new people.
- Having to speak up in public, like at work or school.
- Being easily embarrassed and blushing.
- Looking people in the eye.
- Not knowing what to say in social situations.
- Meeting authority figures, such as doctors and bosses.

If you have social phobia your anxiety is palpable and can lead to utter dread for weeks and months over upcoming events. In fear of anticipated occasions, you may suffer from physical complaints such as breaking out with severe skin problems where you scratch and claw at the sensitive areas, drawing blood. You may have a runny nose, teary eyes, garbled speech, stuttering, gagging, and feel light-headed or faint. Some people use alcohol or drugs to handle the symptoms. Avoidance is a common coping mechanism, which can develop into agoraphobia.

E., Essential

Body dysmorphic disorder is being preoccupied with an imagined physical defect; schizoid personality disorder is a pervasive pattern of detachment from social relationships; pervasive developmental disorder is a type of autism. All of these have major symptoms of social detachment so they must be ruled out for an accurate diagnosis.

What Causes Phobias?

No one knows exactly what causes phobias. There are various theories that try to answer the question, as well as propose treatment solutions. Mental health experts believe that phobias, like other anxiety disorders, are caused by the dynamic mix of biological, cultural, and psychological factors. Since many of the phobias begin in childhood, experts believe they are learned responses, especially specific phobias. Parents may be phobic themselves and pass on the fears, anxious responses, and avoidance behavior to their children. A frightening or traumatic experience with the feared object may occur, for example, being attacked by a dog. Witnessing a traumatic event may also trigger a phobic reaction, for example, seeing someone drown. Having a humiliating experience may also be a cause.

Psychodynamic Theories

Psychodynamic theories vary widely. Many believe that mental conflict, such as anxiety states, are caused by emotions and impulses that are unconscious childhood fantasies and memories, such as loss and guilt. When triggered in adulthood, the person develops anxiety.

Others state that anxiety may develop because of real or feared separation from parents. Unresolved childhood anxiety, for example, the fears in separation anxiety disorder is a cause of developing other anxiety disorders in adult life.

Biological Theories

Biological theories look at recent findings that indicate that abnormalities in certain neurotransmitters such as serotonin and norepinephrine may be the culprits. Others are studying the amygdala, a part of the brain that is linked to emotions, such as fear and anxiety. These researchers are looking for differences or abnormalities in anxious people. Some experts believe that phobias have a genetic basis and inborn traits, such as being self-conscious, shy, and cautious, make one more likely to develop phobias. Mental health experts agree that there is no one reason why you develop a phobia and someone else may not. Another point of agreement is that people and their phobias are complex matters and no simple solution will cure them.

 Alert

Dysthymic disorder is an underlying depressed mood for at least two years. People with dysthmia describe themselves as being sad or blue most days. Other symptoms include low energy, low self-esteem, problems with eating and sleeping, poor concentration, and little interest in life's activities.

Related Conditions

If you have specific or social phobia, you have a high risk of developing other conditions, because these are long-lived persistent disorders that threaten to severely impair your life. Other emotional conditions often appear due to the difficulty in normal functioning or as coping mechanisms to ease the anxiety. These conditions include: depression; dysthymic disorder, which often begins in childhood and is linked to social phobia; panic disorder with agoraphobia; substance abuse; low self-worth; and suicide.

Other physical illnesses and conditions that present especially in social phobia can be severe. Headaches, body pain, stomach ailments, and skin conditions are common. The ability to become independent, have good relationships, marry, and be successful professionally are very difficult to achieve for people with social phobia.

Effects of Gender, Culture, and Family

Phobias are the most common mental disorders. More women than men are diagnosed with specific phobias in the subtypes animal and natural environment. Situational phobias are more often diagnosed in women than men, but the gap is less than in the animal type. The blood-injection-injury type of phobias are also reported more by women. Many studies state that more men seek treatment for social phobia, but others show men and women equal in reporting that disorder. Theories about the gender gap include differences in how men and women are socialized, and the willingness for men and women to seek treatment.

 Fact

The most common reactions of women diagnosed with specific phobias who were afraid of rodents or insects were screaming, avoidance, and asking for help, in that order. Research showed that fewer women were unable to move until the animal was gone.

Cultural differences have to be accounted for when making a diagnosis, and deciding on a treatment plan: understanding religious beliefs, the belief in and fear of magic and spirits, language difficulties, and how women and children are viewed by the specific culture. The diagnosis has to be made using the individual's culture as a frame of reference, as well as determining the degree of distress.

Family patterns indicate that either heredity and learning, or both, are likely factors in the development of phobias. Studies have shown that if parents or other close relatives have specific phobia, animal type, then it is likely that their child or other close relative will have an animal type phobia too, though they may not necessarily be afraid of the same animal. The same statistics hold true for people with situational and blood-injection-injury phobias.

Treatment

Though phobias can be emotionally painful and debilitating and greatly undermine your ability to lead a satisfying life, they are very treatable. Phobias are usually treated with a combination of medication and psychotherapy. The course of treatment usually runs for months, though more severe phobias may take longer. Cognitive behavioral therapy is the most commonly used in treating phobias and helps you to identify and change unreal thought patterns. Exposure therapy teaches you gradual desensitization to the feared stimuli. Stress management/relaxation techniques help you stop the anxious response so you can take control of your anxiety.

Group therapy has also proven an effective method in treating phobias. Groups will help you feel less isolated by your fears, offer support, share coping techniques, and provide a place to learn and practice social skills. Other therapies and methods of treatment include the behavioral types, NLP (neuro-linguistic programming), EMDR (eye movement desensitization and reprocessing), yoga and meditation, diet and exercise, herbal supplements, bodywork, and massage therapies. Many people are treated successfully for phobias without being prescribed medication.

A number of medications are widely prescribed specifically for treating phobias. Antidepressant SSRIs (selective serotonin reuptake inhibitors), particularly Paxil and Zoloft, are considered most effective. Less prescribed are the MAOIs (monoamine oxidase inhibitors), such as, Nardil and Parnate. Benzodiazepines (tranquilizers), which include Xanax, Ativan, and Klonopin, are prescribed to alleviate the severe feelings of anxiety.

Essential

It is important to find a therapy group that is comfortable and is led by a therapist who understands phobias. To find a group contact your physician or local hospital. If you find that the group does not fit your needs, discuss this with your therapist in private, or find another group.

Treatment will be most effective by using a multidisciplinary approach, such as entering individual psychotherapy, starting an exercise program, limiting caffeine, and joining a therapy or support group. But no matter what treatment is decided on, it is up to you to make substantial life changes to help facilitate a "cure."

CHAPTER 5

Obsessive-Compulsive Disorder

Obsessive-compulsive disorder (OCD) is one of the most disturbing and complex anxiety disorders. OCD can manifest itself in a number of ways, and it imprisons its sufferers with mind-bending obsessions and exhausting compulsions, making daily life a nearly impossible challenge. This chapter defines the disorder and details the symptoms, criteria for diagnosis, related conditions, and other relevant information.

Defining Obsession and Compulsion

Both obsession and compulsion make up OCD, so it's important to understand both phenomena and how they work together in those with this disorder. If you are obsessive, intrusive thoughts, ideas, images, or impulses echo again and again in your mind. You realize that the thoughts, images, ideas, or impulses are excessive and inappropriate but are unable to stop them. Being unable to stop the obsessive thoughts may make you feel helpless and hopeless about turning them off or controlling them. The following is an example of obsessive thinking:

> Harry is obsessed with having to know exactly how much change he has in his pocket, especially when he stands in the checkout line in a store. He is terrified that when it is his turn to pay he won't have enough money. Thoughts about not knowing the exact amount of change as he waits in line run rampant in his mind and create severe anxiety. He has dollar bills in his wallet, but that amount does not interest him, for he knows he has enough to pay for what he wants to buy. It is only the amount of the change that drives him wild. He also obsesses about

having to give exact change, and not fumble when he finds out his total bill. Harry feels the mental tapes that play continuously while he's in line are ridiculous. He is fully aware that his obsessive thinking is irrational, but when he tried to stop the counting, his anxiety worsened.

Compulsions are defined as uncontrollable impulses to perform an action or ritual repeatedly in response to an obsession. These actions often have to be repeated in an exact way or the anxiety will increase. The uncontrollable compulsive behavior is a mechanism used to decrease anxiety. Consider the following continuation of Harry's story to better understand compulsion:

To ease his anxiety about the amount of change in his pocket, Harry must count the change. He puts his hand in his pocket and runs his fingers through the coins, counting as he goes. He has been doing this for years and by now can make an accurate count just by feeling the coins with his fingers. Once he knows the exact amount, he feels less nervous. But within seconds, he is questioning the amount, thinking he made a mistake, and worrying about what will happen when he has to pay if the count is inaccurate. The counting is continuous until he pays for his item and leaves the store. Over the years, Harry begins to count change in other situations too; for example, while waiting for his bus to come on the way to work. Sometimes the counting interferes with his job as a truck driver because he has to pull over and count many times during the day, making it difficult to complete his deliveries. There are days when Harry counts change hundreds of times. However, for occasional days at a time, the need to count change eases. Harry is fully aware that change counting is irrational, but when he tries to will himself to stop, his anxiety severely increases.

Harry is obsessed with the change in his pocket and he is compelled to count it over and over again. Most people have obsessive and compulsive qualities, but they generally do not interfere with daily life. If you get extremely anxious and are distressed by recurring thoughts and repeated behaviors similar to Harry's, make an appointment to see your family doctor as soon as possible.

Details of the Disorder

Obsessive-compulsive disorder (OCD) is an anxiety disorder defined as unrelenting excessive anxiety that takes the form of worries, thoughts, ideas, and impulses (obsessions), and the extreme need to control the obsessions by doing a series of ritualistic actions (compulsions). These sometimes frenzied actions make no sense and are time consuming. But if you have OCD you know you must do them to get (temporary) relief from the anxiety. If your compulsion is not accomplished in a "prescribed" manner, there is often a marked increase in your anxiety. You may realize that beneath the bizarre behavior is a generalized fear, usually of some danger to you. The actions or compulsions are an attempt, however ineffectual, to stop these disturbing feelings. It is estimated that about 3.3 million adults, 2.3 percent of the population, have OCD. The disorder can begin in childhood and adolescence.

Criteria for Obsession and Compulsion

The symptoms of OCD inflict severe emotional pain and discomfort, and you can become debilitated in your personal and professional life if you are not treated. Obsessive-compulsive disorder can be difficult to diagnose because obsessions and compulsions appear in many other disorders as well. To begin, you must meet the criteria for obsessive thinking, which includes repeated and invasive thoughts, impulses, or images that you feel are inappropriate, and cause you a high degree of anxiety and distress. These thoughts, impulses, or images are not part of every day problems. You cannot ignore or stop your obsessive thoughts, and are conscious that your thinking comes from your mind and is not created by something external.

To meet the criteria for compulsive behavior you must perform repetitive behaviors, such as hand washing, checking, counting, or silently repeating words without being able to stop them. You must feel compelled to perform these behaviors due to an obsession, or to self-imposed rigid rules. You do these behaviors to ease your anxiety or to stop a feared circumstance from happening. Your behaviors cannot prevent either the anxiety or feared situation and are considered excessive responses.

Essential

OCD differs from other compulsive behaviors such as overeating, abusing alcohol and drugs, and gambling, because these behaviors bring you gratification, at least initially. For example, the gambler may be reinforced by sometimes winning big. But compulsions of OCD are never enjoyable or reinforced with positive results.

Criteria for Formal Diagnosis

To be formally diagnosed with OCD you have to meet the criteria that are laid out in the DSM-IV guidelines. These include:

- You must be aware that your obsessions and compulsions are extreme and unreasonable.
- The obsessions and compulsions must cause you severe distress for more than one hour a day, or significantly disrupt your daily life at work, school, or play.
- Your obsessions and compulsions are not caused by another disorder, for example, being focused on food if you have an eating disorder; pulling out your hair if you have trichotillomania.

Your behaviors cannot be caused by the use of drugs or alcohol, or other mental disorders, such as anxiety disorder due to a medical condition. Your symptoms also cannot be caused by side-effects of medications you are taking in order to be diagnosed. Obsessive-compulsive personality disorder differs from OCD because it involves a persistent pattern of the excessive need to control your environment with perfectionism and starts in early adulthood. Both disorders can be present at the same time.

With varied intensity, OCD affects people in different ways. If you have a mild form of OCD you can live a normal life without too much distress. On the other hand you might suffer from a severe and persistent form of the disorder. Maybe you fall into a third group where your symptoms wax and wane. In trying to describe what it is like to have obsessive-compulsive disorder, individuals state that it is similar to what happens when a record has a scratch in it. The needle gets stuck in the grove the scratch made, and that one note plays over and over again. You may have insight into the fact that your obsessions and compulsions are unrealistic, and that your rituals are weird. Sometimes you are aware that your behavior is excessive, while other times you may see your actions as completely normal.

 Alert

> The extreme intrusive nature of obsessions is called "ego-dystonic," meaning that the person with OCD experiences the obsession as strange and unfamiliar, and out of personal control. Most people with OCD are aware of their behavior, but some are not and, in rare cases, can lose all sense of reality and become delusional.

OCD in Children and Adolescents

Obsessive-compulsive disorder often begins in childhood or adolescence. It is estimated that one in 100 children, or one million children in the United States suffer from it. The average age for symptoms to begin is ten. The symptoms are similar to those experienced by adults, but the obsessions differ. In younger children, obsessive thoughts of being harmed or of parents being harmed or even dying are common. Compulsions to ease these fears are often ritualistic, which can lead to dysfunction at home and school, and with peers.

Children may have a rigid bedtime routine that must be the same each time to prevent an imagined disaster, such as harm coming to their parents. A child might say, "As long as I jump up and down three times, hop on my left foot twice, slap my pillow once in the middle, and turn around ten times to the right before I get into bed, everything will be okay." But if one tiny detail is not done exactly as last time, the ritual begins again until the child can get it right and ease her anxiety. As children with OCD reach adolescence and venture out into the world, their obsessive thoughts and fears change focus from danger to parents to danger to themselves. Getting a disease or having food poisoning is common in teens with OCD. Adolescents may conceal their symptoms due to feelings of shame and will often hide their obsessions and compulsions from peers, parents/family members, and health care providers.

Essential

Mornings and evenings can be very trying for a family with a child who has OCD. If the child's rituals aren't performed perfectly, the child will become anxious and agitated. Children with OCD find it difficult getting to school on time, creating family stress. The evening OCD rituals cut into homework, dinner, and family time. Bedtime may get later making children sleep deprived.

Treatments for Children

Children are treated in much the same way as adults, with a combination of medications and a variety of therapies, such as cognitive behavioral therapy and exposure therapy. In 2003, The Food and Drug Administration (FDA) approved Prozac (fluoxetine) for the treatment of OCD in children and adolescents who are aged from seven to seventeen. Alternative remedies include changes in diet, vitamins, and herbal supplements. Research is ongoing to meet the needs of children and adolescents with OCD.

OCD is a debilitating and often painful condition that makes it very difficult for children to be successful in school and among peers. If your child has OCD, you must educate yourself thoroughly on the best way to help your child and how to cope with your own feelings about your child's condition. These include: getting an accurate diagnosis, understanding what medicines are available and their effectiveness and side effects, finding therapies and alternative treatments, building a support system at home and school, learning good parenting techniques, and finding as many resources as possible.

Typical Symptoms

People with obsessive-compulsive disorder ordinarily display both obsessions and compulsions, but sometimes they may have obsessive thoughts without the compulsions, or vice versa. It is estimated that about 25 percent of people with OCD experience obsessions without the compulsions. Any obsession can be without a compulsion, but the most likely form will be the fear of causing harm to others. In some cases, compulsions do not have obsessions attached to them, but that is more rare.

Common Obsession/Compulsion Pairs

The common obsessions usually have compulsive responses, but the variety of compulsive responses and how they manifest varies for each person. Some typical obsessions and their compulsions include:

- *Fear of dirt, germs, and contamination*: The obsession with cleanliness leads to compulsive cleaning, bathing, and washing. Washing hands hundreds of times a day is common and may become ritualistic, for example, how to specifically wash, or for so many minutes.
- *Worry about having everything "perfect"*: The need to have things arranged in a particularly exact order, for example, the need to have clothes color-coordinated.

- *Fear about harming oneself or others*: Repeated checking of locks on doors, stoves, automobile brakes; having to retrace a driving route for fear you ran over someone.
- *Obsessions about religion*: You may fear that you doubt your belief; compulsive praying.
- *Worry about health*: You excessively check your pulse, follow a rigid diet and exercise routine, and become obsessed about reading the latest medical information.

Other obsessions and compulsions include obsessive thoughts about numbers, words, or sounds leading to compulsive counting or repeating words or phrases over and over. Having forbidden sexual thoughts or urges usually leads to compulsive touching of self or others, or repeated rituals in sexual relationships. Hoarders and savers excessively collect and save objects such as old newspapers, garbage, and animals (often stray dogs and cats).

Not all obsessive-like thinking is associated with OCD. For example, some people like things neat and orderly, religious figures pray daily, and some people call themselves "pack rats." And most people practice daily rituals; for example, eating meals at set times or stopping for a latte every morning on the way to work. It is the degree of behavior and its affect on your daily functioning and life that signals OCD may be present.

Superstitious Fears

One aspect of obsessive-compulsive disorder is the fixation on superstitious beliefs (also called "magical thinking"). If you have severe OCD you are rigid in how you perform certain actions because unless you do it "just so," negative repercussions will occur. Or you avoid doing certain things for the same reason. Superstitious fears and their behaviors include things like avoiding cracks in sidewalks, not crossing certain streets, and thinking that letters, numbers, or colors are lucky or unlucky.

Some people with magical thinking refrain from thinking or saying certain words because they fear some harm will befall them.

Others begin to divide everything in the world into either "negative or positive" and rigidly observe these beliefs in their daily lives. Superstitious fears lead to feelings of dread if the rituals based on the obsessions are not followed. The variety and breadth of rituals is endless and unique for each individual with OCD. Consider Barbara's situation:

> Barbara is in her late thirties and works as an engineer for a construction company. She has suffered from severe OCD since early childhood. Her obsession is that she will get an infectious disease, and she especially fears AIDS. Recently, she moved into a new house and had to throw out a living room chair when one of the movers cut his finger while carrying the chair in, and she saw a few drops of blood on his finger. A number of times she has left a cart filled with groceries on the check out line when she noticed the cashier had a Band-Aid on her finger. It is hard for her to clean her house because she is afraid that touching dirt and dust will make her sick. What is peculiar to Barbara's story is the fact that while she is working on dirty construction sites, dirt and injuries do not bother her. When people get cut or scraped at work, she is not compelled to wash. But at home, she will wash her hands up to a hundred times a day, or shower repeatedly if she brushes up against something that she thinks is dirty. For example, at times when she sees someone with a cut, such as the mover, she does not recognize that throwing out her chair is extreme. She justifies those actions by asking, "Isn't everyone afraid of catching AIDS?" But she is aware that the excessive hand washing is irrational.

Each person suffering from OCD finds ways to justify their odd behavior, which makes the condition somewhat easier to deal with on a daily basis. Of course, the condition always perpetuates itself, and the only way for people with OCD to truly get better is to seek help from a professional.

When and Why Does OCD Begin?

Obsessive-compulsive disorder generally begins in childhood, as early as preschool, or adolescence, but can begin in adulthood, generally no later than forty years of age. The exact causes of OCD are not known. It is thought by some experts that if you have OCD you tend to overreact to anxiety-borne thoughts, because of personality traits. This thinking is the beginning of a vicious cycle, that starts because you are upset by your overreaction, then try to suppress the threatening thoughts. Trying to dodge or bury the thoughts leads to an obsession with that specific thought. When you engage in compulsive actions and feel your anxiety lessen, you are reinforced to repeat the action.

 Fact

Tourette's disorder and tic disorder are thought to be closely connected. In both Tourette's disorder and tic disorder, the person has multiple motor and vocal tics. The tics involve repeated involuntary movement of the head, torso, and upper and lower limbs. The vocal tics are grunts, yelps, barks, sniffs and can involve yelling obscenities, without being able to stop.

Other factors that are suspected in the development of OCD are genetics, as OCD tends to run in families. Studies show a link between having family members with Tourette's disorder or tic disorder and developing OCD. Research also suggests a connection to some infectious diseases such as streptococcal infections, and herpes simplex virus. Biological research is looking at the possibility of low levels of the neurotransmitter serotonin in people with OCD, as well as abnormal functioning of brain circuitry.

Studies are ongoing to determine the causes, treatment, and prevention of obsessive-compulsive disorder. But even without a definite cause, treatment options exist that have shown promise for both children and adults, enabling them to reduce symptoms and lead more productive, satisfied lives.

Diagnosis

If you have OCD you may be seeking relief from the medical community for a long time, as OCD is often misdiagnosed. Studies show that on average, it takes people years, sometimes decades, to be properly diagnosed. Misdiagnosis happens for a number of reasons. For one, you may feel ashamed of your symptoms and hide them or have little insight about your disorder. Also, many health care professionals are unfamiliar with the symptoms of OCD and types of treatment.

The primary tool for diagnosis is an evaluation by a mental health professional that will provide a detailed history of the obsessive and compulsive symptoms, the severity of the condition, and information about possibly related conditions. Both a neurological and cognitive examination will also be performed.

Related Conditions

Obsessions and compulsions appear in many other conditions, making proper diagnosis of obsessive-compulsive disorder very difficult. Since people with OCD may not be forthcoming about their condition in therapy, it is important for the health care clinician to ask pertinent questions to elicit the information. Other related conditions that a health care professional considers when making a diagnosis include:

- Tourette's disorder
- Tic disorder
- Epilepsy
- Head injuries
- Substance abuse
- Schizophrenia
- Previous streptococcal or herpes infections

The health care provider will also look for signs of major depression, and other anxiety disorder, eating disorders, somatoform disorders, and impulse disorders, such as kleptomania and trichotillomania, to be able to provide education to you and your family and to set up an effective treatment plan.

Effects of Gender and Culture

Obsessive-compulsive disorder is diagnosed equally in men and women and is found in every socioeconomic and ethnic group. Cultural norms will play a large part in determining if someone has OCD.

 Fact

At one point, OCD was thought to be rare, but more than 100 million children and adults suffered, or currently suffer, from OCD worldwide. The World Health Organization lists OCD as one of the top five worldwide conditions and the fourth most common mental disorder after phobias, substance abuse, and mood disorders.

Researchers doing cross-cultural studies have found distinct differences in obsessions. In Western culture, cleanliness, health concerns, and sexual obsessions predominate. In Middle Eastern countries, religious obsessions predominate. The recent focus of cross-cultural studies and other research is to find a universal biological cause of OCD.

Treatment

Treatment for obsessive-compulsive disorder is comprehensive and combines medication, psychotherapy, education, and family support and is based on severity of symptoms, awareness of patient to his or her disorder, whether another disorder or condition is present, and other specifics in the person's evaluation. Using medication to alleviate OCD is successful, with 50 to 70 percent of people with OCD responding positively. The FDA has approved a number of antidepressants for treatment of OCD that include: clomipramine, fluvoxamine, paroxetine, sertraline, and fluoxetine.

Research indicates that traditional psychotherapy has not shown great results in treating OCD, but behavior therapy has. One type of behavior therapy, also called exposure and response prevention, has shown to be effective in reducing OCD symptoms when combined with medication. Similar to desensitization treatment for phobias, exposure and response prevention exposes the individual to the feared object or idea either in reality or imagination and then discourages or actually prevents the person from responding with compulsive behaviors. For the therapy to be most effective, the person must be motivated and the family must be involved in treatment. Research shows that by combining medications and behavior therapy, the majority of OCD individuals are able to function well in daily living.

Essential

Though many OCD sufferers respond well to medications, the side effects can be rough. They include drowsiness, dry mouth, constipation, nausea, sexual dysfunction, headaches, gastrointestinal problems, tremors, diarrhea, dizziness, apathy, and anorexia. Even more radical treatments are used for those with severe OCD who are resistant to standard treatment. These include neurosurgery, and electroconvulsive therapy (ECT).

CHAPTER 6

Stress Disorders

Experiencing traumatic events can change your life and have a serious effect on the way you relate to family, friends, and the world at large. Your ability to cope with and transcend terrifying and life-threatening experiences will determine your chances of developing one of the stress disorders. There are two of these disorders: post-traumatic stress disorder and acute stress disorder. This chapter will cover manifestations of these disorders, criteria for diagnosis, related conditions, and treatment options.

What Is a Stress Disorder?

The stress disorders, posttraumatic stress disorder, and acute stress disorder are defined as the development of debilitating anxiety and other severe symptoms following a traumatic event, either one that you have personally experienced or witnessed. The experience is either a real or symbolic life or death situation, a situation that can end in either serious personal injury, or threaten your nature and being. The main characteristic of stress disorders is having feelings of extreme fear, horror, and helplessness at what is occurring, and then experiencing recurrent mental images of the event that frighten and disturb you. The kinds of incidences that can lead to the development of a stress disorder include terrorist attacks, military combat, and rape.

Shell shock was changed to many other names, including neurasthenia, battle exhaustion, nervous exhaustion, hysteria, and battle shock. Later, the medical community realized that these symptoms also applied to anyone who had experienced traumatic events, and in 1980, the stress disorders were included in the DSM-IV.

 Fact

> Prior to the term postttraumatic stress disorder, the term "shell shock" was used during World War I to describe the specific mental symptoms soldiers suffered due to physical causes, specifically, the effects of an explosion, or of being buried by an explosion. Eventually, shell shock came to describe all the emotional symptoms associated with combat.

Posttraumatic Stress Disorder (PTSD)

The criteria for the stress disorders are similar, but there are important variations that call for making a correct diagnosis and for putting together an effective treatment plan. The DSM-IV lists seven areas of criteria that have to be met for making the diagnosis for PTSD. Mental health practitioners should be aware that individuals suffering from PTSD may have difficulty reporting their symptoms and talking about the events that led to their problems, so gentle but probing questions are important during the initial evaluation. Criteria for diagnosing posttraumatic stress disorder are as follows:

- You have experienced or witnessed events where there was a possibility of death or serious injury, or death occurred, or you or someone else was threatened emotionally.
- You felt intense fear, horror, and helplessness during the event.
- You re-experienced the trauma by recollections, images, thoughts, or perceptions of the event. You have reoccurring disturbing dreams of the event, or relive the trauma through feelings, hallucinations, and dissociative flashback episodes.
- You feel physiological and psychological distress when faced with anything that reminds you of the event.

You may also chronically avoid anything that provokes associations with the trauma, and experience numbing in your thoughts, feelings, or conversations about the event. Avoidance of people, places, or activities that remind you of the event is common. You may be unable to recall details of the event and have little or no interest in life activities. You may feel detached and estranged from others and believe that your life has no future (e.g., relationships, career, living long). Sleep problems, increased irritability, and angry outbursts are common, as well as difficulty concentrating. You can become hyperalert and wary and develop a magnified startle response. Symptoms must be present for at least one month, and they must create intense distress and disrupt significant areas of functioning in your personal relationships, work, and school.

There are three specifiers for PTSD used for diagnostic purposes. Specifiers indicate when the symptoms began and how long they have been present. Acute specifier is used when the symptoms are present for less than three months. The chronic specifier is employed when symptoms last for at least three months or longer. And with delayed onset, at least six months have passed between the trauma and the beginning of PTSD symptoms.

Essential

Children with PTSD make sense of the trauma differently than adults. They may engage in repetitive play that expresses the content and details of the trauma. Children may have nightmares but are often not able to connect dream content to the trauma. If reminded of the trauma, physical and emotional symptoms may appear.

Acute Stress Disorder

Acute stress disorder, like posttraumatic stress disorder involves the development of severe anxiety and other acute symptoms in response to a traumatic event. The symptoms begin either immediately or within one month. The major difference with posttraumatic stress disorder is that in acute stress disorder the symptoms must peak and be alleviated within one month. If symptoms persist, then a diagnosis of PTSD is given as long as all criteria are met for that disorder. By specifying the differences between acute stress and PTSD, mental health clinicians are able to plan a proper treatment program.

Question

What does dissociation mean?
Dissociation is a cognitive process whereby a person disconnects from his feelings, thoughts, memories, and sense of self, as a way to cope with a traumatic event or situation, while it is occurring or after the trauma is over. The experiences of losing touch with one's present surroundings can range from mild, such as "daydreaming," to the serious dissociative states of PTSD.

The diagnosis for acute stress disorder includes the presence of dissociative symptoms such as derealization, depersonalization, and dissociative amnesia. You have to re-experience the event in flashbacks, thoughts, dreams, and hallucinations. Other symptoms include anxiety, sleep problems, irritability, depression, and an increased startle response. You may avoid anything linked to the trauma, and experience severe distress in your personal and professional life. However, none of your symptoms can be caused by brief psychotic disorder, or the physiological effects of medication or abuse of drugs or alcohol.

Understanding Stress Disorders

The basis for understanding the stress disorders is the ability to comprehend the complex nature of trauma. If you have experienced a traumatic event or situation, you may or may not develop a stress disorder. If you do, your symptoms may be mild and transient, or severe, and last for years. A number of external factors about the event, including the characteristics and previous experiences you have had, will often determine the prevalence and course of the disorder. The external factors depend on the seriousness and length of time the trauma continues, as well as the extent to which you were exposed to the event or situation.

Trauma is a profoundly disturbing experience, either of a severe physical injury or emotional shock. Whether trauma is experienced due to a physical and emotional event, such as war or rape, or a completely psychological situation, such as losing your job or being sexually harassed, there are common aspects of trauma. These include the situation coming as a surprise or shock, inability to change or handle the situation, and an inability to stop the situation from occurring. Trauma is a unique experience, and a disturbing event that will emotionally level one person may not have the same effect on another. Your response to trauma and your risk of developing a stress disorder depends on many factors. If you do develop a stress disorder, it is not a sign of weakness and requires proper diagnosis and treatment as soon as possible.

The Physiological Response to Trauma

Researchers on stress disorders who study the physiological process of psychological trauma have studied a number of factors that might explain why trauma persists in memory, sometimes for years, along with "flashbacks." One is that there is abnormal activity in the amygdala, which releases stress hormones when there is danger, and is a factor in the depth and longevity of the memory of emotional trauma. Others are studying what happens when people disconnect from the instinctual "fight or flight" response. In psychological trauma there is often a numbing of emotions from the event and that may be the reason why your body cannot return to its normal balanced state. Researchers believe this numbing leads to a higher risk of developing PTSD.

Some people with trauma have abnormal levels of certain hormones, like norepinephrine, which is released during a stress reaction. Norepinephrine activates the hippocampus, the part of the brain involved in storing information in long-term memory. Researchers continue to look for preventative strategies and treatments to stop or heal the symptoms of stress disorders.

 Fact

In 1977, psychologists Brown and Kulick studied traumatic recurring memories, calling them "flashbulb memories," by questioning people on their experiences when they heard that President Kennedy was assassinated. They theorized that during unusual and shocking events a specific component of the brain activates and "freezes" the traumatic moment, like a camera takes a snapshot—called a "Now Print."

How Stress Disorders Progress

Stress disorders usually develop over a period of days or weeks following the traumatic event. Individuals who have chronic PTSD may have periods when symptoms increase, due to other stressors or reminders of the trauma, followed by a lessening of symptoms. Some people experience unrelenting symptoms, while others report mild symptoms that spike occasionally when memories of the event arise. Your vulnerability, previous experiences, present stressors, personality traits, coping mechanisms, support systems, and whether you have another emotional disorder could play a part in the development of PTSD. For example, individuals who were raped or sexually molested as children seem to have a higher probability of developing a stress disorder in adulthood. But if you do not have high risk factors and experience a traumatic event, you may also develop PTSD.

Additional Symptoms of Stress Disorders

If you develop a stress disorder your symptoms can range from mild to severe and take weeks, months, or years to heal. Sometimes symptoms begin months after the event, making it difficult for you to relate your anxiety and discomfort to the trauma. The following are other symptoms of stress disorders:

- Anxiety and panic attacks
- Depression, sadness, crying, feelings of despair
- Low energy and fatigue
- Eating problems (loss of appetite or overeating)
- Sleep problems (insomnia or sleeping too much)
- Chronic pain or achy joints
- Sexual dysfunction
- Feelings of numbness or indecision
- Development of obsessive-compulsive behaviors

Present research shows that some "flashbulb memories" remain in astonishingly accurate detail decades after the trauma, but studies indicate that many traumatic memories can fade over time or be distorted in their accuracy. Experts believe that it is important to study the degree the trauma provoked the individual psychologically, as well as other factors to understand trauma's staying power.

Traumatic Events and Situations

One of the major factors in determining if you will or will not develop a stress disorder is how you experience or witness the trauma, how you interpret it, and how you feel about the events or situation. The events that often lead to acute stress disorder or posttraumatic stress disorder have common features that include a real or perceived life and death situation, severity and length of trauma, and situations that are beyond human control or comprehension. These events and situations are numerous and range from military combat and torture, to rape and being the victim of a robbery. Experiencing natural or man-made disasters, being in a severe automobile accident, having a permanent debilitating injury, being diagnosed with a serious or terminal illness, and being the victim of hate crimes also lead to PTSD.

The events leading to the beginning of a stress disorder do not have to be the more common life-threatening ones as listed above. New research looking into stress disorders is studying experiences, such as discrimination, sexual harassment, bullying, and a build up of stressful experiences over time as other possible causes of stress disorders.

Essential

Complex PTSD results from succeeding negative stressful events, such as domestic violence and persecution. Though usually not life-threatening, these situations have characteristics that include feeling isolated and trapped, loss of power and control, having boundaries violated, and being rejected and humiliated.

Who Develops Stress Disorders?

Anyone can develop a stress disorder, and it can develop at any age, from early childhood into late adulthood. Some people are more vulnerable, for example, children or people who are dealing with other significant stressors, like poverty. It is estimated that approximately 8 percent of people in the United States will experience PTSD at some point in their lives, and that twice as many women as men will develop PTSD. Studies have shown if the trauma includes rape, that population, which includes men, women, and children, has the greatest likelihood to develop posttraumatic stress disorder. Besides enduring physical violence, the victim may also fear being judged, stigmatized, not believed, and rejected by family, friends, and society, which increase vulnerability for developing PTSD.

Women and Stress Disorder

Women face being violently victimized in our culture more often than men. Women are victims of rape and other types of violence, such as domestic violence and stalking, more often than men. High numbers of females develop PTSD, double that of men. Statistics show that over 90 percent of attempted rapes and 89 percent of rapes were against females, twelve years and older. All rape victims, regardless of gender, experience serious mental and physical symptoms. The most common experiences women have in the development of stress disorders besides rape are being sexually molested and physically attacked or threatened with a weapon, childhood physical abuse, and domestic violence.

Men and Stress Disorders

The most common experiences for males who develop stress disorders are being in combat, rape, molestation, neglect, and physical abuse in childhood. Men who work as firefighters and other rescuers who face traumatic events on a regular basis often develop stress disorders. Though they have chosen their line of work, are well trained, and debriefed after a disaster, sometimes the build-up from seeing many disturbing experiences and the magnitude of an event will make coping extremely difficult. After the attacks of September 11, 2001, rescuers reported difficulty getting in touch with their feelings, had increased anxiety, problems sleeping, nightmares, and increases in irritability and anger. The rescuers at the Oklahoma bombing site who were more likely to develop PTSD were those who spent more hours and days going through the rubble looking for the remains of victims.

Military Combat

Many soldiers who return from war come home with more than physical injuries and have a good chance of developing a stress disorder. Soldiers returning from Iraq will face the same adjustment other veterans have experienced in previous wars, finding it difficult to leave the images and memories of combat behind them, and pick up their lives prior to war.

The Veterans Administration is already preparing for the influx of new vets facing stress disorders. Like in Vietnam, the Iraq war is being fought against guerrillas, and that kind of warfare increases feelings of vulnerability and the risk for posttraumatic stress disorder. As of the summer of 2004, 20 percent of returning soldiers from Iraq have sought mental health care, and about 17 percent of those suffered from PTSD symptoms or the full-blown disorder. Common symptoms soldiers may experience are: symptoms of depression; cutting off from loved ones, and feeling comfortable only with other vets; having an exaggerated startle response, for example, hearing a car backfire and running for cover; and mentally replaying images of battles or dead comrades. Those with physical injuries have a very high probability of being diagnosed with a stress disorder as well.

Fact

Approximately 1.7 million Vietnam vets have been diagnosed with PTSD, mostly unrelated to physical injury. The longevity of PTSD was seen in 1994, when veterans of World War II reported a return of PTSD symptoms on the fiftieth anniversary of D-Day.

Research into the treatment of returning vets indicates that the majority of soldiers who need help do not ask for it. One reason is that if they have PTSD they are numbed out and shut off emotionally from the trauma, hide their symptoms, and are afraid of being stigmatized and seen as "weak."

Children and Stress Disorders

Children and youth are an especially vulnerable group and can develop stress disorders at early ages. Whether they have to cope with being separated from or losing a parent, family instability, being sexually molested, being involved in an accident, or having to cope with a serious illness, young children may experience symptoms that include: recurring memories of the event, nightmares, worry about dying, loss of interest in usual activities, behavioral problems, heightened startle response, age regression, and physical complaints. They may also develop separation anxiety from parents or guardians, and cry, scream, whimper, and regress developmentally. Older children and teens may also manifest substance abuse, defiant or violent behavior, and not want to leave home to go to school. If a child was physically or sexually abused, they may act out the abuse by becoming abusers themselves.

Families and Stress Disorders

It's not just the victim of the trauma who suffers and needs help dealing with the significant changes that have taken place, but families can show signs of stress disorders too. These difficulties include:

- Families may feel emotionally and physically cut off by the member who experienced the trauma and has lost the ability to trust.
- The victim may feel numb, unable to show emotion and affection.
- Family members may feel rejected by the victim.
- The victim may lose interest in family activities.
- Both family members and victim may be afraid to discuss the trauma.
- The family may become angry or frustrated when the victim doesn't return to "normal" functioning quickly.

Essential

Your psychological characteristics may place you at higher risk of having severe reactions to trauma. If you have low self-esteem or a pessimistic outlook on life, trauma may be difficult to handle. Being diagnosed with dependent personality disorder or borderline personality disorder places you at risk for stress disorders, as both are characterized by feelings of low self-worth, the need to be taken care of, and poor life coping skills.

Examples of these situations may include: a returning soldier being unable to emotionally engage in holiday festivities, or be attentive to his loved ones, creating anger and resentment from family members, or a rape victim being unable to resume sexual relations with her spouse who feels rejected and angry.

Related Conditions

Individuals who are diagnosed with posttraumatic stress disorder or acute stress disorder often have other physical and emotional conditions. Some of these conditions are coping strategies to help them handle the trauma, while others develop because of the body's reaction to severe stress. The related conditions include emotional conditions such as depression or major depressive disorder, which develops in more that 50 percent of people diagnosed with posttraumatic stress disorder. Panic disorders with agoraphobia, social and specific phobias, and obsessive-compulsive disorder often present after a trauma.

 Fact

Research shows that a high percentage of women with PTSD also abuse drugs and alcohol. Alcohol is most commonly abused followed by cocaine and marijuana dependence. Studies indicate that individuals who use drugs and alcohol as a coping mechanism for PTSD symptoms have difficulty learning other coping skills and take longer to work through the trauma.

Somatization disorders that are characterized by complaints of pain, gastrointestinal distress, sexual problems, and other symptoms that significantly disrupt, but are not due to a medical condition, are commonly linked to stress disorders. Survivors of trauma have a high risk of suicide or attempts for a number of reasons that include: developing depression, feeling helplessness and hopelessness, feeling guilty for surviving, and not being able to control or stop the trauma. As an example, people who were raped may feel damaged and guilty, believing they are at fault for the assault, or that somehow they could have stopped it.

Severe stress compromises the immune system and survivors of trauma are open to developing diseases, such as heart and lung diseases, cancer, high blood pressure, gastrointestinal illness, and skin conditions. Substance-related disorders commonly occur as a way of "self-medicating" to cope with the trauma.

After a trauma has occurred it is difficult to determine if other mental or physical conditions developed before or after the traumatic event. The initial interviews for diagnosing stress disorders must include detailed mental and physical health histories. And treatment planning must take into account the need to remedy the coexisting disorders as well as the presenting stress disorder.

Assessment and Treatment

Stress disorders, especially PTSD, are conditions that require professional help and treatment. Research shows that if you are assessed and treated as soon as possible after trauma, you are less likely to develop a stress disorder and other conditions, and if you do, you have a better chance of recovery. Your first step in treatment is with your family physician, who will examine and test for physical conditions. It is crucial that you be referred to mental health professionals, such as psychiatrists, and psychologists, who can properly diagnose you for a stress disorder and develop an effective treatment plan. The mental health practitioner will do a detailed initial evaluation and ask for information such as:

- Personal and family history
- Mental and physical health history
- General information about your personality and coping style and skills
- Previous drug and/or alcohol use
- Previous traumas and how you reacted
- Details about the present trauma

Your mental health clinician will rule out other medical conditions, such as head injuries, and mental conditions, such as personality disorders, and use the DSM-IV as a guide in making a diagnosis of either acute stress disorder or posttraumatic stress disorder.

Fact

Tests and assessments tools used to diagnose and plan treatment include questionnaires, such as the Mississippi Scale for Combat-Related PTSD, Impact of Event Scale, the Veronen-Kilpatrick Modified Fear Survey, and the Children's Impact of Traumatic Events Scale. Tests that look at the person's progress during treatment include The Beck Depression Inventory.

Stress disorders are complex conditions and treatment is multifaceted. Though there is no known cure, a combination of psychotherapy and medication has shown to be effective in relieving symptoms and helping to develop coping skills. Cognitive therapy that involves connecting to the trauma and working through it can help you change how you cognitively process the emotions of the trauma. Behavioral therapy teaches relaxation exercises and desensitization to distressing stimuli. The most common medications prescribed are the antidepressants, Zoloft and Paxil. Benzodiazipines, such as Xanax, Ativan, and Valium, may be prescribed to treat the anxiety and phobias that accompany stress disorders.

Chapter 7

Generalized Anxiety Disorder (GAD)

Generalized anxiety disorder is quite common, though it is estimated that less than a quarter of people with GAD are treated. A person who suffers from generalized anxiety disorder spends much of their time excessively worrying about the daily routines of life and how others view them. The worrying cannot be stopped and intrudes on personal and professional functioning. This chapter covers the basics of this often disabling anxiety disorder, and how it is assessed and treated.

What Is GAD?

Generalized anxiety disorder is a disorder that affects children, adolescents, and adults. It was included in the DSM-III in the 1980s. GAD is more prevalent than panic disorder and specific phobia. If you have generalized anxiety disorder you most likely find it very difficult to function in daily life. Generalized anxiety disorder is recognized by its main characteristic: excessive apprehension and worry about almost everything you do or are involved in. You also worry about family members, friends, and coworkers, with no way to turn off the distress and worry. If you have GAD, you experience many symptoms including concerns about how others view you, and how you will be evaluated on your performance in many aspects of your life. If you have GAD, you always feel that disaster is right around the corner.

What Does Generalized Mean?

The word "generalized" means to spread widely. In GAD, the term applies to the pervasiveness of the worry and anxiety into everything that makes up your life. The anxious feelings associated with GAD are often not connected to a particular thing, person, or situation and are considered a "free-floating" anxiety that comes seemingly out of nowhere for no known reason. But the worry can be directed to past experiences and upcoming situations and events too.

 Fact

Generalized anxiety disorder (GAD) affects 4 million to 5 million people in the United States. There's an 8 to 9 percent chance that a person will develop it in the course of a lifetime. GAD affects more women (60 percent) than men (40 percent); 30 percent of people with GAD will be diagnosed with panic disorder, and an equal number with depression.

Criteria for Generalized Anxiety Disorder

The symptoms relating to generalized anxiety disorder are chronic and create pain, suffering, and significant impairment in daily living, while also impacting family members. The following must be met for diagnosis:

- You experience worry and anxiety that is greatly out of proportion to events and circumstances for at least six months.
- You cannot stop or control the worry.
- You experience symptoms such as restlessness, fatigue, and difficulty concentrating.
- You are irritable.
- You have muscle tension.
- You have trouble sleeping.
- You worry your distress significantly impairs your life.

For diagnosis, these symptoms cannot be caused by either another anxiety disorder, medical condition, or substance abuse. Frequently people with GAD have other anxiety disorders, such as panic disorder, depression, substance-induced anxiety disorder, and somatic complaints, such as dry mouth, nausea, diarrhea, and a startle response, making a diagnosis very difficult.

Doesn't Everyone Worry?

If you always worry about everything, you may assume everyone else does too. The truth is everyone worries sometimes. Some people thrive on stress and worry, and working or living under pressure. But people with generalized anxiety disorder worry to excess and often have feelings of obsessive thinking, dread of mistakes made in the past, or upcoming events, fears of being in certain situations to be rated and evaluated. These emotions create severe anxiety, which interferes with the ability to perform normal activities. Generalized anxiety doesn't mean that you will necessarily avoid situations, but if most of your time is given over to excessive thinking and concern, then you may become incapacitated from doing anything else. Most often your fears aren't caused by any one thing; there's no sense of cause and effect.

Essential

Generalized anxiety disorder (GAD) may last for twenty years, with low rates of remission and moderate rates of relapse after remission. The progression of GAD is influenced by a number of factors, including gender, stressful life events, and sensitivity to anxiety. A diagnosis of GAD must have already ruled out possible medical causes.

Physical and Emotional Symptoms of GAD

Perhaps you are aware that your feelings are irrational but can't help yourself. You may experience any or all of the following physical and mental symptoms: headaches, shakes, twitching, feeling unstable, irritability, lack of concentration, frequent urination, nausea, vomiting, diarrhea, and trouble swallowing. And because the obsessive thinking is unrelenting, you can begin to feel hopeless about your situation.

GAD and Agoraphobia

There is a correlation between GAD and the development of panic disorder and social phobia. If that occurs then agoraphobia may develop too. If you chronically worry that you will say the wrong thing, spend hours obsessing about what you did say, think that people are negatively evaluating you, are terrified that you will make a mistake, and the hundreds of other concerns you have, then avoiding situations that create such severe tension is understandable. If you do begin to avoid people, places, and things that frighten you, full-blown agoraphobia may develop. Avoidance offers a little relief for the moment, but since GAD anxiety is mostly not situation specific, the chronic worry will not be alleviated.

The Effects of GAD

Generalized anxiety disorder is a chronic disorder, but symptoms can range from mild to severe. It seems the external stress and other conditions increase the severity of symptoms, and they may remain high for long periods of time if you do not seek treatment. Consider Jane, a GAD sufferer, and her situation:

Jane is in her mid-twenties, single, living alone, and a college graduate. Jane has been anxious since she was a child, but her symptoms decreased during her middle and high school years. After graduating from high school, moving into her own apartment, and getting a job at an insurance company, Jane's symptoms gradually increased and are now severe. Jane is keyed up all the time, sleeps poorly, is exhausted, and has not been able to concentrate at work; stays late almost every night. She worries all the time that she will be fired. She has begun avoiding meetings and contact with co-workers whenever she can because she feels like a failure.

Without treatment Jane's condition will only worsen and may incapacitate her, negatively impacting her career.

Causes of GAD

There are a number of theories about what causes the development of generalized anxiety disorder. Researchers and theorists continue to study why such severe worry and dread begins often in childhood, becomes chronic, and continues into adulthood, sometimes with little let up of symptoms. The three main theories come from biological theory, genetics, cognitive behavior theory, and psychological theory.

Biological theory looks at a number of areas: that the amygdala that controls emotion is turned on and does not shut down, producing anxious responses to life events. Researchers are also studying the reactivity in the autonomic nervous system, neurotransmitter levels like serotonin, and other areas in the brain such as the hypothalamus, thalamus, and limbic system.

Genetics examines how the disorder is passed on to family members and research indicates that it plays a role in GAD. Studies show a frequency with members of the same family having the disorder, but studies on twins show little difference between identical and fraternal twins.

Cognitive behavior theory states that it is the individual's reactions to stimuli that he deems threatening and dangerous that causes the development of anxiety disorders. Cognitive behaviorists believe that the person with anxiety has a distorted view of what constitutes danger to themselves, as well as a belief that they are incapable of coping and cannot control the situation—leading to anxiety symptoms.

Psychoanalytic theorists believe that anxiety develops because of unresolved unconscious conflicts from childhood involving libidinal gratification, the id, ego, and superego. Other psychological theories suggest that unresolved issues that come from childhood are based on experiences and repressed emotions such as anger and rage.

Though you may have a "tendency" based on biological, genetic, and other causes to develop GAD, it's not certain that you do. It may take external events and stressors such as a major life transition to "trigger" the start of the disorder. These high risk factors include high stress at work or school that you cannot cope with, problems with intimacy or relationships that include love interests, family members, friends, teachers, and employers. Loss of employment and financial problems create high stress and worry. If you have sleep problems and other health conditions, you may be vulnerable to developing GAD.

Fact

A correlation exists between general anxiety disorder and depression, phobia disorder, and panic disorder. GAD usually develops during adolescence, though most people wait until adulthood before seeking treatment. Getting GAD after age twenty is not uncommon. It is a lifelong disorder in most people.

Life Disruption

If you are suffering from generalized anxiety disorder you may feel that you have little life outside of your excessive worry and foreboding. You never feel at ease about anything, cannot calm down, have difficulty concentrating and making decisions, and worry about misfortunes that you know are sure to come. Suffering includes many symptoms such as tension headaches and feeling jittery and having your mind go blank making it difficult for you to work, go to school, be in crowds, and enjoy life. Your apprehension covers everything you think about or do, and you may have trouble with the following:

- Romantic relationships and friendships
- Sexual intimacy
- Communication problems
- Avoidance issues
- Family relations

People with generalized anxiety disorder miss more work than those without the disorder. GAD affects productivity and advancement in the workplace, and people with it can have panic attacks and phobias making it difficult to attend business meetings, give presentations, travel, and interact with important business contacts. It's no wonder that people with GAD often can't get ahead at work and worry that their jobs are in jeopardy.

If you have GAD, your distress and excessive worry make it very difficult for you to put things in perspective. For example, you may become terrified that your friend has died in a car accident if she is three minutes late for lunch. Parents with GAD often act out in anxious ways if their children are a few minutes late coming home, or a husband may get frightened and then very angry if his wife is late coming home from work, even if it was unavoidable. GAD is an enormous burden on the person dealing with it, but it also has a far-reaching impact on friends and family.

Essential

Generalized anxiety disorder was first introduced in DSM-III-R in the 1980s. In the current edition, DSM-IV, published in 1994, GAD was changed from a catchall category describing persons who don't fit other anxiety categories to a well-defined condition.

GAD and Children

Children and adolescents, like adults, are under a lot of stress and pressure and experience anxiety sometimes on a daily basis. Talk to any kid and you will hear worries about friends, parents, grades, teachers, sports and coaches, clothing, body image, blemishes, love, etc. But the worries and concerns a child with GAD has are of a different nature with more intense emotions, and manifesting a host of symptoms. If your child's worries become excessive and begin to disrupt his or her life as well as yours, then you may be looking at a diagnosis of GAD. Generalized anxiety disorder begins in childhood anywhere from age five up to late adolescence, and symptoms often change as the child reaches adolescence.

Fact

Approximately 50 percent of generalized anxiety disorder begins in childhood or adolescence. It is aggravated by any stressful situation that heightens fears already held by the individual, such as fear of inferiority, fear of insecurity, fear of rejection, fear of illness and death. GAD is associated with mood disorders and psychotic disorders.

Symptoms in Children

Almost the same criteria are used for diagnosing children and adolescents as adults, but a child's or adolescent's fears and worries are different than those of adults. Their fears center around the safety of themselves, family and home, their ability to perform well at school and in athletic events, upcoming events where they may be uncomfortable and afraid, and natural disasters or events out of their control, like hurricanes. Some children become obsessed about being on time. Others do not want to go to school, won't visit friends or go to sleepovers, and may cling to parents. Many children need constant reassurance to keep the anxiety under wraps. Adolescents may use drugs and alcohol to self-medicate, become truant, and avoid socializing with their peers.

Children suffering from GAD will experience some physical symptoms, including stomach aches, headaches, fatigue, irritability, muscle aches, tightness in throat, sleep problems, stomach problems, nausea, rapid heart beat, and trembling. Children with GAD suffer intensely, have problems interacting with peers, and have a difficult time growing emotionally.

Treatment for Children

Research and studies show that the most effective form of treatment is cognitive behavioral therapies. The cognitive work includes: educating children on their disorder, helping them become aware of their negative self-talk and irrational beliefs, and teaching children to change them. The therapist will help children become alert for physical signs that anxiety is building, and teach them effective coping strategies. Behavioral techniques include breathing and relaxation, guided imagery and systematic desensitization. Family therapy that targets communication, management of anxiety, and problem solving is an important component for treatment.

 Alert

There is considerable cultural variation in how anxiety is expressed. In some cultures anxiety is expressed predominantly through physical symptoms, in others, through mental symptoms. It is important to consider the cultural context when evaluating whether worries about common situations are excessive.

Medication is also an option. The most commonly prescribed medication for children are the SSRIs. Prozac has been prescribed to children for years, but Paxil and other SSRIs are being prescribed too. A recent warning by the FDA regarding the risk of suicide in children who take SSRIs has not stopped the drugs from being prescribed, as some doctors feel that the benefits outweigh the risks. But they are on alert for problems.

Helping Your Child with GAD

There are a number of ways you can help your child and at the same time ease your own stress and tension about your child, as well as create a calm environment for the whole family. Work on increasing your child's self-esteem and confidence so she feels capable of coping with the anxiety. Curb your frustration and disappointment when your child cannot do things that other kids can. Teach your child to relax. In fact, make it a family project so the whole family feels better. Work on lessening perfectionist behavior by teaching your child to set realistic goals, and to use failures as a learning experience. Emphasize positive self-talk and the use of affirmations.

 Fact

According to the National Institute of Mental Health, a diagnosis of depression, or other anxiety disorders, may make developing GAD more likely. The individual with generalized anxiety is consumed by the "what ifs." As a result, there's no way out of the vicious cycle of anxiety, apprehension, and worry, and the person inevitably becoming depressed about the situation.

Related Conditions

There are many mental and physical conditions that contribute to the development of generalized anxiety disorder, and conditions that appear alongside it make diagnosis and treatment planning difficult: depression is common in people with GAD, and other anxiety disorders found in people with GAD are obsessive-compulsive disorder (OCD), panic disorder, phobias, and posttraumatic stress disorder (PTSD). Many people with GAD may also have a major mental illness such as schizophrenia. Drugs and alcohol are commonly used to self-medicate, but other substances like caffeine in high doses may be involved in its development. Withdrawal from drugs like cocaine, marijuana, benzodiazepines, and antidepressants may cause GAD symptoms.

Other conditions that may be associated with GAD are irritable bowel syndrome (IBS), frequent headaches, asthma, and hyperthyroidism (Grave's disease). Because of the severe tension involved, teeth grinding and insomnia are also common.

Diagnosis and Treatment

Like other anxiety conditions, generalized anxiety disorder can be difficult to diagnose because its symptoms mimic those of other disorders. Your doctor will gather information through diagnostic interviews with you, your child if he or she is the patient, and other relevant family members. Your physician will have to know your family medical history, and any pertinent information about symptoms, addictions, behaviors, major changes or life transitions, and traumas. Your doctor may use assessment tests, such as Diagnostic Interview Schedule for Children (DISC), the Multidimensional Anxiety Scale for Children (MASC), and the Screen for Anxiety Related Emotional Disorders (SCARED) for adult or child. By using the DSM-IV as a guide, your doctor will make a diagnosis and set up a treatment plan.

Treatment for GAD is either medication or therapy, or a combination. The most common drugs prescribed are quick acting benzodiazepines, such as Xanaz, Valium, Librium, Klonopin, and Ativan. These are highly addictive and meant for short-term use to ease severe symptoms. The side effects of benzodiazepines are drowsiness and problems with balance. Antidepressants can be effective and the SSRIs like Prozac and Zoloft are often prescribed. They have side effects too and can take weeks to take effect. BuSpar is another drug utilized for GAD.

Alert

People taking benzodiazepines who wish to suspend the medication are urged to taper off to prevent seizures, delirium, and death, which may occur if the drug is suddenly stopped. For more information, read the drug's packaging material and speak to your physician.

Cognitive and behavioral therapies are highly effective in helping you change your patterns of thinking and behaving. Relaxation and systematic desensitization are taught to increase anxiety symptoms and increase coping skills. Psychodynamic therapy helps you become aware of feelings and learn healthy ways to express them. Family therapy, group therapy, and use of support groups are other effective treatments. Alternative treatments include massage, diet and exercise, and stress management.

CHAPTER 8

Anxiety Due to a Medical Condition and Substance-Induced Anxiety

Numerous medical conditions, diseases, and syndromes include anxiety as a complicating symptom, but these conditions can also lead to the development of an anxiety disorder, such as panic disorder or generalized anxiety disorder. Additionally, the use of stimulants, drugs, and alcohol, or withdrawing from them, may lead to the development of a substance-induced anxiety disorder.

What Is Anxiety Disorder Due to a Medical Condition?

The main feature of anxiety disorder due to a medical condition is that the severe anxiety and resulting impairment must be directly due to the physical effects of a medical condition, such as hyperthyroidism. The anxiety cannot be caused by how the individual feels about the disease—anxiety must develop due to the physical results of the disease. For example, the anxiety cannot begin because you are upset about having the disease. If that is the case, then the mental health provider would diagnose the person with adjustment disorder with anxiety, meaning that you are having difficulty "adjusting" to a life stressor. Diagnosing for mental health disorders is difficult and this disorder can be especially tricky. The criteria for diagnosis include:

- You have severe anxiety from panic attacks, generalized anxiety, or obsessions and compulsions.
- Medical exams, tests, and your medical history show that your anxiety is directly related to a general medical condition.

- Your symptoms are not caused by another mental condition or delirium.
- Your symptoms create severe emotional disturbance or disruption in your life.

The clinician making the diagnosis must also be sure that another anxiety disorder, such as obsessive-compulsive disorder is not the cause of your distress before diagnosing you. This will ensure proper diagnosis and treatment.

Medical Conditions That Cause the Disorder

The number of medical conditions, diseases, and syndromes that may lead to an anxiety disorder is so numerous that only the most common will be discussed in this book. Cardiovascular diseases cause heart arrhythmias, heart attacks, blockage of blood vessels, and can produce anxious symptoms, such as chest pain, difficulty catching one's breath, and feelings of dread and apprehension. Thyroid diseases can lead to heart palpitations and anxiety symptoms. These include: hyperthyroidism, hypothyroidism, and thyrotoxicosis. Alzheimer's/dementias are progressive neurodegenerative diseases that often cause fear and anxiety in the early stages. Cushings' syndrome is a disorder of the adrenal glands that causes excessive secretion of cortisol, a stress hormone, leading to symptoms of anxiety. Mitral valve prolapse is a slight defect in one of the heart valves. It is harmless but can cause heart palpitations, chest tightening, and breathlessness. Both premenstrual syndrome and menopause cause hormonal changes and often anxiety symptoms. Hyperventilation creates symptoms similar to panic attacks, such as dizziness, shortness of breath, shakiness, and depersonalization.

Other diseases and conditions that are strongly linked to anxiety are: metabolic conditions, such as diabetes; Meniere's syndrome or disease, an inner ear disturbance; lung diseases such as emphysema, epilepsy, and other seizure disorders; and obstructive sleep apnea. Vitamin deficiencies and allergies to foods or the additives in foods, as well as properties in medications may lead to symptoms of anxiety. Poisons like pesticides and cleaning fluids may cause dizziness and rapid heart beat and, with long exposure, can lead to anxiety disorders.

 Fact

Complex B vitamins play a vital role in healthy brain function. For example, niacin has been shown to sustain brain cells and mental sharpness. B vitamins also aid in the production of neurotransmitters, which help regulate mood, and send messages between the brain and other parts of the body.

Diagnosis and Treatment

Your doctor will begin by evaluating for a known medical condition, or one that you may be unaware you have, with a physical exam and laboratory tests. Taking a detailed personal, family, and medical history will help your doctor determine if a primary anxiety disorder exists. If you are taking medications, other substances, herbs, supplements, etc., your doctor will want to rule out other conditions, such as substance-induced anxiety disorder, by having you take a blood drug screen, and urine analysis. Your doctor has to ascertain whether your anxiety can be explained by the stress of having the medical condition. One important guideline is examining the timing of the onset of the medical condition and the symptoms of anxiety. If your physician cannot determine that the anxiety was a direct cause of the medical condition, or find another diagnosis, then a diagnosis of anxiety disorder not otherwise specified may be given.

Treatment for the anxiety symptoms must be coordinated with the physician treating the medical disorder, especially if anxiety medications are prescribed. Treatment will depend on the type of anxiety symptoms specified when the diagnosis is made. A combination of psychotherapy and medication is usually recommended, depending on the severity of the symptoms. Traditional psychotherapies that are effective in treating anxiety include cognitive, behavioral, dynamic therapies, or a combination, depending on reported symptoms. You may be prescribed antidepressants, such as Paxil, or anti-anxiety medications like Xanax, and sedatives such as Restoril.

Basics of Substance-Induced Anxiety Disorder

The main characteristics of substance-induced anxiety disorder are significant symptoms of anxiety that are caused directly by the effects of a substance. Substances might include alcohol, recreational drugs, medication, or exposure to a toxin. Your symptoms may appear either while you are using the substance, or develop during withdrawal. The criteria for diagnosis includes:

- You must suffer severe anxiety, panic attacks, or obsessions and/or compulsions.
- Your history, physical exam, and laboratory results prove that the substance is the cause of your anxiety.
- Your anxiety is not caused by another anxiety disorder.
- Your anxiety cannot develop during delerium.
- Your symptoms have to significantly impair your life.

The diagnosis can be made only when the symptoms are more severe than those usually associated with substance intoxication or substance withdrawal, and when the anxiety requires separate clinical treatment.

Essential

When either anxiety disorder due to a medical condition or substance-induced anxiety disorder is diagnosed, a specifier is attached to it describing the type of symptoms the person is experiencing. Specifiers are any of the following: generalized anxiety, panic attacks, obsessive-compulsive symptoms, or phobic symptoms.

Symptoms may develop during the person's use of the substance, if so, then the specifier used is "with onset during intoxication." If the symptoms begin during or shortly after withdrawal of substance, then the specifier is "with onset during withdrawal." The specifiers help mental health experts design an effective treatment plan.

Substances That Cause the Disorder

There are nine categories of substances that include stimulants such as cocaine; sedating substances such as alcohol and sleeping pills; hallucinogens like LSD and marijuana; inhalants, such as glue and spray paint. Over-the-counter or prescribed medications that may cause anxiety are antihistamines, antidepressants, insulin, oral contraceptives, and cardiovascular medications. The category called "other" (unknown substance) is used when the substance cannot be identified.

Sedatives

Sedatives are drugs that depress the central nervous system (CNS) and cause calmness, sleepiness, diminished anxiety, slower breathing, and slow, uncertain responses. Sedatives are called by a number of names that include: tranquilizers, soporifics, anxiolytics, depressants, sleeping pills, downers, and sedative-hypnotics. At high doses many of these drugs can cause unconsciousness and death. Sedatives are used by doctors as anti-anxiety agents, anti-epileptics, muscle relaxants, and for medications before the delivery of anesthesia.

When taken for an extended period of time, all sedatives can cause dependence, even at therapeutic doses. When dependent users seriously cut back or suddenly stop taking the drug, they will show withdrawal symptoms ranging from restlessness, insomnia, and anxiety to convulsions and death. When users become psychologically dependent, they exhibit the intense surety that they need the drug to get by, although there is no biological dependence. In both instances, dependent users go to great lengths to get the drug and use it. Though they can be abused, sedatives play their rightful role helping people.

Fact

Sedative-hypnotic drugs are given intravenously (IV) but are also administered orally. These drugs depress behavior, moderate excitement, induce calmness, and cause drowsiness. They are used clinically as anti-anxiety agents, muscle relaxants, anti-epileptics, and as pre-anesthetic medications.

Alcohol

Alcohol is a sedative and thus depresses the central nervous system. Initially, it acts as a stimulant, but more drinks lead to sedating effects. In small quantities alcohol relaxes, lowers inhibitions, slows reflexes, and decreases concentration and physical coordination. In moderate amounts, effects might include slurred speech, drowsiness, and mood changes. Large amounts of alcohol cause vomiting, difficulty breathing, unconsciousness, coma, and death.

Stimulants

Stimulants that affect the central nervous system are a broad based category of drugs whose characteristics produce feelings of euphoria, alertness, and a sense of well-being. Many stimulants come from natural sources, others are produced in labs. Legal stimulants are prescription-only controlled substances or over-the-counter products, and some are also illegal. Stimulants include amphetamines, and amphetamine-like substances, cocaine, caffeine, and nicotine.

Amphetamines

Amphetamines and amphetamine-like substances are a group of drugs that are a combination of chemicals that are artificial stimulants. The basic drug is amphetamines, also known as, uppers, bennies, and pep pills. Other drugs in the group are called dextroamphetamines and methamphetamines, known as speed, crystal meth, crank, and ice. Amphetamines can be taken orally in the form of pills, sniffed in crystal or powder form, injected, or smoked.

When users experience the feelings of euphoria, they may go on "binges," to maintain the good feelings. After smoking or injecting amphetamine, an immediate, intense rush of pleasurable feelings occur, which last for only a few minutes, making the user wanting to keep the high by immediately using again. Amphetamines affect the brain, as well as the heart, lungs, and other organs.

Essential

Amphetamines were first used in the 1930s to treat narcolepsy, which is an inherited sleep disorder characterized by falling asleep without warning. It was added to nasal sprays, which was discontinued, but later used as a treatment for depression, weight loss, and attention disorders.

Methamphetamines and Ecstasy

Methamphetamines are the most powerful of the amphetamines, and have a stronger effect on the nervous system, making them highly addictive. Methamphetamines are controlled substances that require a doctor's prescription but are also produced illegally and sold as street drugs. The effects of "meth" can last for up to eight hours and after the initial "rush," usually lead to a state of intense agitation, and at times violent behavior. Amphetamine users feel a temporary boost in self-confidence and power, but those feelings can quickly change when the effect of the drug wears off, or they stop using. Users become dependent on the drug to avoid the "down" feeling experienced when the drug's effect wears off.

The stimulant 3.4-methylenedioxymethamphetamine (MDMA), commonly called Ecstasy, is popular and notorious for its misuse during date rapes and similar offenses. MDMA has the effects of euphoria, high energy, and social disinhibition, which last three to seven hours.

Amphetamine-related psychiatric disorders occur most commonly in white individuals. With intravenous use, amphetamine-related psychiatric disorders occur three or four times more commonly in males than females. With nonintravenous use, amphetamine-related psychiatric disorders occur equally in males and females.

Cocaine

Cocaine is a powerful stimulant, derived from the coca plant, native to South America, and has been used for thousands of years by indigenous tribes. In the 1850s, scientists synthesized the leaves into a white powder, and by 1880, cocaine was being used in medicine as a surface anesthetic.

Initially, cocaine was thought to be a wonder drug and was used in everything from tonics to toothache cures, as well as an additive to wine and soft drinks. It was widely used by the American public, and stores sold chocolate cocaine tablets. But by the early 1900s the addictive nature of cocaine and its other dangerous side effects were beginning to be recognized. When the Dangerous Drug Act of 1920 was passed, cocaine was on the list.

Fact

Cocaine has a storied past. Sigmund Freud used it himself and prescribed it to his patients as a cure for depression and sexual impotence. In the 1890s, Coca-Cola skyrocketed to the number one soft drink in America because its main ingredient was cocaine, which produced euphoria, and consumers felt energized by drinking it.

Cocaine is usually "snorted," inhaled as a powder, and quickly enters the bloodstream. There is an initial "rush" and feeling of well-being, and feeling energized and more alert and open to your surroundings. But the high doesn't last long, and on the way down, the user may feel very depressed. Wanting to maintain the "high," or keep away the depression leads to abuse. Long-term use leads to the build up of a tolerance for the drug, so more and more is needed to feel the euphoria.

When cocaine powder is heated into a liquid, and the fumes are inhaled through a pipe, the concentration of cocaine entering the bloodstream is very high. Called "freebasing," these high doses can severely strain the cardiovascular system and cause death. Crack is more addictive than other forms of cocaine, and users can be hooked after the first use. If alcohol is mixed with cocaine, the liver combines the two substances into a new one, called, cocaethylene, which heightens the euphoria, but increases the risk of sudden death.

Nicotine

Nicotine is a powerful drug and comes from the tobacco plant, nicotiana tabacum. Tobacco was first introduced into Western civilization in the 1500s, but Native Americans, and peoples in other parts of the world, such as Asia, were using it long before that. Native Americans used it as a curative for physical and mental afflictions.

L. Essential

In 1965, the U.S. Congress enacted a law that required all cigarette packages to carry the warning that smoking may cause lung cancer, and lung and heart diseases. It is presently estimated that more than three million Americans die of medical conditions from the direct effect of smoking.

Nicotine, an alkaloid, is the substance that causes the addiction and its side effects. At high doses nicotine is toxic, but at low doses it has medicinal qualities. When you smoke a cigarette, the nicotine almost immediately enters the lungs, then the bloodstream, and in about eight seconds it reaches your brain. When tobacco is chewed, nicotine enters the bloodstream through the mucous membranes of the mouth, or if snuff is used, it enters through the nose.

Nicotine affects the central nervous system and has both positive and negative influences on the body and emotions and can be either anxiolytic, which means it lowers feelings of anxiety, or anxiogenic, meaning it increases anxiety. The down side of nicotine includes respiratory problems, hypertension, vomiting, seizures, gastrointestinal problems, and an increase in anxiety and depression. The positive side of nicotine is an increase in cognitive function; it can create painlessness without numbness; it protects cells in the nervous system from damaging diseases; and it widens blood vessels in the brain.

Hallucinogens

Hallucinogens (psychedelics) are a group of drugs that alter perceptions, thought, awareness, and emotions. They have a long history of use. Many cultures have used and still use hallucinogens for religious purposes. Hallucinogens include such drugs as lysergic acid diethylamide (LSD), the first synthetic hallucinogen, psilocybin, DMT, and mescaline. Some hallucinogens are natural, such as mescaline from the peyote cactus; others such as LSD are synthetic. LSD was discovered in 1938. It is one of the most powerful mood-changing chemicals. LSD is sold on the street in tablet form, capsules, and sometimes as a liquid. It is usually ingested orally, but sometimes it is injected.

Fact

The highest rate of hallucinogen abuse occurs in persons aged eighteen to twenty-five years. According to the 1996 National Institute of Drug Abuse high school student survey, hallucinogens are the third most frequently abused class of drugs by high school students, after alcohol and marijuana.

The effects of psychedelics are unpredictable and depend on the amount taken. The first effects of the drug begin thirty to ninety minutes after taking it. The physical effects include dilated pupils, raised body temperature, increased heart rate and blood pressure, sweating, and tremors. Sensations and also perceptions change. And hallucinations and delusions occur. All these changes can be frightening and can cause panic. Having a bad psychological reaction ("bad trip") to LSD is common.

Most people who take hallucinogens never go for medical help unless they've taken a massive overdose. Individuals who seek medical intervention probably do so because of a bad trip and are disturbed by visual hallucinations and acute anxiety.

Cannabis

Cannabis, also known as marijuana, is an illegal drug that comes from the dried leaves and flowers of the Cannabis sativa plant. Other names and forms of cannabis include: hashish, pot, weed, and dope. THC (tetrahydrocannabinol) is the active ingredient that causes the "high." Cannabis is usually smoked but can be eaten. THC is a potent ingredient that alters the brain and is linked to the development of anxiety disorders. When smoked, it enters the bloodstream quickly through the lungs and moves immediately to the brain. The "high" usually lasts for a number of hours, depending on the strength of the drug, and the person's size, health, and emotional state. Cannabis may stay in the body for days, even after only one dose. The immediate effects of marijuana include:

- Feeling a sense of well-being
- Laughter and becoming talkative
- Having difficulty concentrating
- Loss of coordination

Craving food, having an increased heart rate, and bloodshot eyes are other symptoms. If you consume large amounts of cannabis, the effects may be negative and include feelings of being paranoid and confused, becoming restless, experiencing feelings of unreality, and having anxiety and panic attacks. Cannabis is not physiologically addicting like nicotine, but psychological dependence occurs when the drug becomes part of one's lifestyle.

Phencyclidine (PCP)

PCP and similar substances were originally created in the 1950s for use as anesthetics that were injected intravenously. By the mid-1960s, these drugs were no longer in use due to the severe side effects, but because of the intense "high" they produced, they became street drugs. Today, PCP is manufactured illegally and sold under the names angel dust, rocket fuel, ozone, and wack. PCP is a powder that is formed into tablets, capsules, and colored powders, to be ingested, snorted, or smoked. If it is smoked, it is often combined with herbs like mint and oregano. If marijuana is the additive, then the combination is called either "killer joints" or "supergrass." Some users smoke menthol cigarettes dipped in liquid PCP called "super-cools," "hydro," "wet," and "fry." PCP quickly enters the brain and is highly addictive. Prolonged use can lead to cravings and compulsive behavior in trying to obtain it, dissociative states, feelings of being invulnerable, exaggerated feelings of strength, and numbing of mental functions.

 Alert

PCP users often end up in hospital emergency rooms due to overdoses or exhibiting violent behavior and are a high risk for suicide. In 2003, it was reported that 2.3 percent of the U.S. population aged twelve years and older have used PCP at least one time. Repeated use is mostly found in individuals aged twenty-six years and older.

PCP's physiological effects are a rapid increase in breathing and pulse rate, rise in blood pressure, numbness in all extremities, and loss of motor control. People who use PCP for long periods of time suffer from memory loss, cognitive defects, anxiety, and depression. In very high doses nausea and vomiting occurs, along with blurred vision, uncontrollable eye movements, loss of balance, and dizziness. Blood pressure and respiration drops may lead to seizures, coma, and death.

Inhalants

The group of substances called inhalants is comprised of hundreds of ordinary household and commercial products such as glue and spray paint. These products are made up of solvents, gases, and nitrites. Products used as inhalants include solvents such as paint thinners, dry cleaning fluids, degreasers, gasoline, glue, correction fluids, some felt-tip markers, and cleaners for electronic devices. Also included are gases in butane lighters, propane tanks, whip cream aerosols, refrigerant gases, spray paints, hair or deodorant sprays, ether, chloroform, and nitrous oxide (laughing gas). Nitrites are (cyclohexyl nitrite) found in room deodorizers; amyl nitrite used in medical procedures; and butyl nitrite, which was used in antifreeze and perfumes (it is now classified as an illegal substance).

Fact

Studies show that generally the first use of inhalants occurs between late childhood and early adolescence. A 2003 National Survey on Drug Use and Health reported that about 23 million people in the United States aged twelve (eighth grade and older) have used inhalants at least once. Other surveys show that 1.3 percent of twelve- to seventeen-year-olds report present use.

Inhalants are ingested through "sniffing" or "huffing," which is done by inhaling the substance through the mouth. Sniffing or huffing is accomplished by either directly inhaling from the container, by putting a plastic bag over one's head and sniffing the fumes, or sniffing a cloth that has been saturated with the substance.

The "high" from inhalants is intoxicating but only lasts for a few minutes. There is an initial feeling of being stimulated and longer use results in feelings of being less inhibited and out of control. Continued use may cause unconsciousness. Sniffing the high concentrations in aerosols, butane, and propane may lead to heart failure and death because the inhalants take the place of oxygen in the lungs and central nervous system, leading to death by suffocation. This is called "sudden sniffing death" and may occur after only one session of inhaling.

Treatment

Both anxiety disorders due to a medical condition and substance-induced anxiety disorders are complex conditions and difficult to treat. The family physician will do a detailed medical exam and run a battery of tests and then refer out to a mental health specialist, usually a psychiatrist. The mental health specialist will do a detailed interview of personal, family, and medical history and use his or her experience and the DSM-IV as a guide to make a proper diagnosis. If a diagnosis involves a medical condition, the physician will continue with any medications for the medical condition and may add medications to alleviate the anxiety. A referral for psychotherapy to a counselor or psychotherapist may be made.

Substance-induced anxiety disorder will require blood tests and urine analysis. Treatment will require the user to stop taking the substance. Depending on the level of addiction, many users will have to go through a detoxification and rehabilitation program. The psychiatrist will also set up a treatment program that may include medication such as anti-anxiety or antidepressants, and psychotherapy like cognitive-behavioral therapy. Attending support groups, such as Alcoholics Anonymous (AA) is often recommended as part of the treatment, as well as including the family in educational and supportive programs.

Chapter 9

Separation Anxiety Disorder (SAD)

Many children have difficulty leaving home to go to school, staying with relatives while their parents are away, or sleeping over at their friends' houses. This separation from home into the greater world can cause extreme distress for these children and their families and, if not treated, may lead to the development of other anxiety disorders. This chapter focuses on separation anxiety disorder and its criteria, onset, and treatment.

What Is Separation Anxiety Disorder?

As children grow and try to make sense of the world around them, fearing things like the dark and strangers is common. Feeling anxious and insecure is a healthy response for a child to show when the adults the child has become attached to leave the child's presence. From infancy to about age four, separation anxiety is considered normal child development, and the child's behavior usually consists of being clingy and crying but will usually pass if the child is gently refocused on something else or comforted. This ability to recognize and miss being with mommy and daddy is called "object permanence." After that developmental period, if a child begins to show signs of extreme distress and anxiety when leaving the parent or guardian, then separation anxiety disorder may be developing.

Separation anxiety disorder is a common disorder and is characterized by excessive anxiety about being separated from parents or any person the child is attached to or being away from home. It begins before age eighteen. The average age of onset is 7.5 years, but the disorder has a specifier, "early onset," that indicates SAD before six years of age. Avoidance manifests in behaviors such as refusing to go to school or not wanting to stay over at a friend's house. Symptoms may go into remission but exacerbate during major life events or transitions, and the disorder can last into adulthood.

Object Permanence

Object permanence is a term from Jean Piaget's theory on child development. In Piaget's sensorimotor stage (birth to two years), babies recognize "mother" but are not aware that "mother" exists once she is out of sight. At about eight months old, the child begins to differentiate between "self" and "mother" and in that stage achieves object permanence, that people and things continue to exist even when they are not present.

Ages for Separation Fears

In the normal course of child development, separation fears manifest at eight months, twelve months, and between eighteen months to three years. Separation anxiety generally shows up at around nine months and peaks between twelve to twenty-four months. Separation anxiety generally decreases between two and three years of age. The degree of difficulty the child has may vary from day to day, with one day being more independent and another being clingy and sad. As a child grows there is more of a drive toward independence, but transition times may cause a start in separation symptoms.

Essential

It is estimated that in the United States, separation anxiety disorder (SAD) affects as many as 4.7 percent of children from ages seven to eleven, and 1.3 percent of teenagers from fourteen to sixteen years old. Separation anxiety disorder affects about 2.4 percent of the world population.

Criteria for SAD

The symptoms experienced by children and adolescents who have separation anxiety disorder become chronic and cause mental suffering. These expressions of anxiety can cause significant impairment in your child's daily life as well as create stress, anxiety, and conflict in your family. Your child must meet the following criteria for a diagnosis of SAD:

- Has excessive anxiety in anticipation about leaving home or parent.
- Fears that death or disaster will occur to a parent when the child is away from home.
- Reluctance/refusal to go to school or be away from home.
- Afraid to be alone without a parent.
- Afraid to go to sleep without parent next to her.

Fact

A consideration that clinicians and researchers need to have in understanding child mental health and illness concerns the importance of age and timing. For example, a behavior that may be quite normal at one age (e.g., young children's distress when separated from their parent) can be an important symptom or indicator of mental illness at another age (e.g., separation anxiety is not normal for adolescents).

Other symptoms include recurring nightmares about being separated from parents, fears of animals, monsters, burglars, fear of the dark, tantrums, and numerous physical complaints, such as stomach aches, headaches, and vomiting. Your child experiences extreme distress and disturbance in social, academic, and other important areas of functioning. The disorder is not caused by other mental disorders including autism, schizophrenia, or psychotic disorder and does not meet the criteria for panic disorder with agoraphobia.

What's Wrong with My Child?

Many children express their emotions around major life transitions, like beginning school, with fear reactions. It's hard for many children to leave the safety and comfort of parents and home and go to school where there are strange kids who may not like them, and adults who have different expectations than their parents. School is a place with a new set of rules where a child will be evaluated, graded, and judged against her peers.

If you have a child with separation anxiety disorder, the anticipation of leaving home to go to school may exacerbate the symptoms by the child clinging to you, following you around the house, crying, and not being able to sleep days before the big day. Getting your child to school and then leaving her there may become a frustrating and embarrassing event if your child clings, screams, and sobs while other children seem to have no problem. This scenario might repeat itself for a few days and, as your child adjusts, separating might become easier. However, separation anxiety could also develop into a chronic disorder, increasing your child's suffering and negatively impacting your family.

 Alert

In the United States, one in ten children and teens has serious emotional and behavioral problems. Many others have symptoms that may lead to problems that will grow more serious if the individual is not seen and cared for by a professional. It is important that the child not think that the problem is hers alone, or her fault.

Physical and Emotional Symptoms

Depending on the age of your child, he or she may be unaware that the fears are irrational. Older children and teens most likely are aware, but stopping the feelings and reactions to separation seems impossible. Symptoms include: panic attacks, heart palpitations, stomach aches, dizziness, headaches, nausea, vomiting, diarrhea, crying, worry, anger, acting out (tantrums), refusal to go to school and to participate in other activities, inability to fall asleep without a parent present, and nightmares.

The symptoms of separation anxiety disorder often lessen, and the disorder may go into remission and then reappear during stressful events or times of life transitions. But SAD may become chronic and last into adulthood or eventually develop into panic disorder either with or without agoraphobia. Specific phobias and social phobia may also develop.

Symptoms Found in Age Groups

The symptoms associated with separation anxiety change as your child matures developmentally. Children eight years old or younger tend to have unrealistic worries about harm to their parents and school refusal. Children aged nine to twelve years are more likely to feel distressed in situations like friend's sleepovers, school trips, and sleep-away camp. Adolescents between twelve and sixteen years show more fears around school refusal and physical complaints, such as headaches, dizziness, sweats, lightheadedness, or stomach ache, nausea, cramps, vomiting, muscle and body aches.

Causes and Effects of SAD

A number of reasons and theories exist to explain the development of SAD. Genetics seems to play a role because children diagnosed with SAD are more likely to have a family member with an anxiety disorder. Some research connects children with SAD to mothers who have panic disorder. Learning most likely plays a role as children observe their parents who have attitudes about going out into the world, and model poor coping skills in dealing with life stressors.

It is believed by experts that separation anxiety disorder can develop from a major life transition or a significantly stressful or traumatic experience at a young age, which includes: loss of parent through divorce, a long separation because either the parent or child is hospitalized, the parent is in jail, or away because of military duty, etc. Other experiences are moving and going to a new school. Trauma such as physical, sexual, and verbal abuse, witnessing violence, and being a victim of war or natural disaster may bring on SAD.

Biological theories are looking into chemical imbalances in levels of serotonin and norepinephrine, as well as other hormones and respiration. Some researchers are studying influences during pregnancy such as endocrine release. Others are looking at what happens to children when they lose or are separated from the parent in infancy and brought up by someone else—these studies show a strong link to development of anxiety symptoms, depression, and learned helplessness. Numerous causes exist for the development of separation anxiety disorder and treatment plans must look at biological, genetic, psychological, and environmental factors.

The effects of having a child with SAD can be difficult to cope with. It is heartbreaking to watch your child suffer, but at the same time you may feel afraid, frustrated, annoyed, angry, disappointed, and exhausted. If your child has SAD, he or she will most likely take up a great deal of time and attention. Children with SAD often need constant reassurance if a separation is imminent. Siblings may feel resentful or ashamed of their sibling's behavior. You may argue with your spouse about your reactions and responses to your child's behavior, and maybe even blame each other. Your child may not develop emotionally in a healthy way because of the fears, or go on to develop other anxiety disorders. But professional help, proper diagnosis, treatment, and education can make a positive change.

 Fact

Among those children who enter treatment, SAD is equally found in both boys and girls. Some surveys indicate the disorder is more common in girls (DSM-IV). The diagnosis should also take into consideration children and teenagers who live in dangerous neighborhoods and have reasonable fears of leaving home.

Risk Factors

There are many factors that lead to the development of separation anxiety disorder that include environment, the child's personality, and parenting. You may have an anxiety disorder or a close family member may make your child more likely to be at risk for SAD. Your child's temperament plays a part; maybe he is shy and more sensitive to stimuli, and certain events can trigger the disorder.

Parenting plays a part in the following ways: by being extremely close or even enmeshed and unknowingly not teaching your child how to cope with growing up and entering the world. And some parents reinforce separation anxiety by not being firm about separating when the child doesn't want to. Examples are allowing your anxious child to stay home from school (encouraging avoidance) while not giving the child a chance to learn how to cope with the anxiety. Also, giving your child more attention in the form of comforting, enabling, yelling, etc., when your child is refusing to separate than when they are not. Not comforting the child is a tough line to walk but it is better than enabling and reinforcing behaviors you do not want.

Essential

Adults with separation anxiety disorder are typically overly concerned about their offspring and spouses and experience marked discomfort when separated from them. The disorder limits these individuals from the ability to deal with change in their circumstances (e.g., moving, jobs, vacation, divorce).

Additional Risk Factors

Additional factors that may create conditions for SAD to develop have to do with family environment and routines. When your child is going to have to separate from you or the house, try to have your child rested. Being overtired and cranky will make it harder for your child to cope with the situation. Children with SAD are sensitive so changes in your household routine may disturb your child. A stable structure will make your child feel safe. If major changes or traumas occur, such as the birth of a sibling or a change in caregiver, learn how to deal appropriately in a way the child can understand at their developmental stage.

Ways to Decrease the Risk of SAD

Examine your own behavior and that of family members for enabling and reinforcing behaviors. Socialize your child by modeling that leaving home is okay (watch for your own anxiety about separating from home or doing new things). Bring a babysitter in (when your child is about six months) so the child gets used to you being away and he can feel okay with other caregivers; start with a few hours and gradually increase time. Set up play dates at around twelve months, and eventually get involved in a play group by age three. You may want to enroll your child in preschool a few days a week to encourage leaving home and expand socialization skills. Expect the symptoms and behaviors to continue for a while and learn how to cope with them.

Helping Your Child Avoid SAD

There are a number of things you can do to reduce the chances of your child developing separation anxiety disorder. It's best for you to talk this over with other adults who will be interacting with your child so you can be sure of consistency between the child and the adult caregivers.

- Never make fun of your child's fears, or punish him in any way because of separation anxiety. And do not allow family members to tease or ridicule your child either.
- Never just drop your child off at a new place or with a stranger without taking time to help him get used to new environments and people. Put a positive spin on the experience.
- Allow your child to take something special from home. Called a "transitional object," something like a stuffed toy can represent you and the security of home while he's away.

- Be loving and understanding but firm about guiding your child to separate by assuring him that he will be okay.
- Don't make a big deal out of leaving and remind him that he'll always come back home again later.
- Do not use bribery to force behavior.

Above all, listen to how your child feels, but also point out when he has handled a situation well. The praise he receives for being brave will boost his confidence.

Related Conditions

There are a number of mental disorders and conditions closely associated with SAD. Major depression may be present and symptoms of feeling sad and helpless are common. Studies show a link between SAD and the development of panic disorder with agoraphobia into adulthood. Anxiety disorders such as posttraumatic stress disorder may develop if the child has been abused or experienced other traumas. If the child has suffered a devastating loss of a parent or caregiver, symptoms might be related to grief. Unresolved loss or trauma may lead to chronic underlying depression, called dysthymia. Social phobia and specific phobia have similar criteria to SAD and may be present.

New situations such as the first day of school may be associated with an adjustment disorder. Learning difficulties like attention deficit disorder, and dyslexia, or being placed in an inappropriate academic level may make school, and other situations like it, very difficult for your child to navigate. Situations that may exacerbate or lead to separation anxiety disorder include violence in school or the neighborhood, teasing and bullying at school, or having a physical disability or injury. Older children may have problems with drugs or alcohol.

Diagnosis

Separation anxiety disorder can be difficult to diagnose because the symptoms of the disorder are similar to other conditions and there may be complicating factors such as trauma. The assessment will include a complete medical history and physical exam to rule out medical conditions that include: mitral valve prolapse, diabetes, anemia, lead poisoning, and thyroid problems. Interviews will take place with your child to find out about his symptoms. The clinician is likely to assess for suicide ideation if the disorder is severe. Interviews with all family members may be necessary to obtain family history of anxiety or other mental disorders. Other caregivers may be asked to provide information if school refusal is an issue, for example, teachers. The clinician will need to know when your child's symptoms began, their development, and in what situations your child is struggling to aid in diagnosis. Clinical information regarding family dynamics is important to assess if the interactions with your child are unwittingly increasing your child's anxiety.

Other assessments include a comprehensive family interview assessment that examines family dysfunction and communication styles. The clinician will want to find out if precipitating factors have occurred such as losses, major life transitions, or traumas. Family patterns of relating to one another are important to determine what dysfunction is present, for example, if the child and parent are enmeshed.

Essential

When making an assessment for separation anxiety disorder, cultural differences must be taken into account. Cultures vary in regard to the value they place on interdependence of family members and what time frame is normal or abnormal for children to begin separating from parents and home.

Treatment

Treatment for separation anxiety disorder is often a combination of psychotherapy, both individual for the child and family therapy, medication, and education about the disorder, its course, skills for helping child, etc. Cognitive behavioral therapy will help your child with behavioral techniques that include systematic desensitization, teaching you the principles behind positive reinforcement, and exposure therapy. A cognitive therapist will work on helping your child to adjust and adapt to the feared situations through changes in thought patterns and behaviors. Psychodynamic psychotherapy can help your child work through feelings, become aware of his reactions, and set out a plan to make positive changes. Family therapy will help family members become aware of dysfunctional patterns of communication and behavior and learn ways to guide the child to independence as well as learning how to communicate and express emotion in healthy ways.

Medications most likely prescribed for separation anxiety disorder are the selective serotonin reuptake inhibitors (SSRIs), such as paroxetine (Paxil) and venlafaxine (Effexor), have been shown to be effective in reducing symptoms of separation anxiety disorder, but they do not have approval from the U.S. Food and Drug Administration (FDA) for children under twelve years of age. And recent warnings have been posted that SSRIs may cause an increased risk in suicidal ideation in children and adolescents. Benzodiazepines such as Xanax have been used to treat children, but for no more than two to three weeks due to side effects and possibility of addiction.

Helping your child cope and manage the distress of separation anxiety disorder can be frustrating and difficult. But with comprehensive assessment, proper diagnosis, and a multidimensional treatment plan that includes education, therapy, and medication if indicated, you have a good chance of getting your child on track to grow developmentally and separate to take his place in the world.

Alert

Early treatment of SAD can prevent future difficulties for your child as he moves along developmentally. Without treatment your child will most likely have feelings of low self-worth and may be unable to develop friendships, fail to reach social and academic potential, and continue to suffer with anxiety throughout his life.

CHAPTER 10

Causes of Anxiety

Anxiety is a complex human condition, and anxiety disorders, which create physical, mental, and emotional distress, have no known single cause. Experts do agree that a combination of internal and external factors is at play in the development of anxiety disorders. Studies are being done to understand the relationship between these factors. This chapter covers the popular theories about anxiety, why your personality counts, and how medications, physical illnesses, and other causes can trigger anxious reactions.

Heredity

Your genetic makeup determines nearly everything about you, from hair color, to body type, to what diseases you are prone to, your attitude, behavior, and even your emotions. Most experts agree that heredity is a component in anxiety disorders—maybe in some disorders more than others. For example, panic disorders seem to run in families. Research into the connection between genetics, anxiety, and the interaction of other factors is ongoing, and a number of findings have been made. Researchers who studied obsessive-compulsive disorder (OCD) found that 35 percent of people with OCD, which constitutes 2 to 3 percent of Americans, had a close relative who had the disorder, too. Researchers isolated a number of genes that might make someone prone to OCD, for example, the gene called catechol-O-methyl transferase.

The Gene Connection

In the late 1990s, German researchers stated that they had found the gene that contributes to how much an individual worries. The versions of the gene were involved with serotonin levels: with one type of gene more serotonin was produced; with the other the levels of the hormone decreased. Researchers estimate that the genes being studied would account for 4 percent or less of anxiety disorders, and that other factors, such as environment, play important roles. Other recent genetic studies include Pet-1, a gene that scientists believe controls levels of aggression and anxiety. Though the studies were done on mice, researchers are hoping to eventually test people for Pet-1 variations. And studies of identical twins who have panic disorder showed that genetics is a factor in that disorder, but that environmental factors were as important.

Twin Studies

Twin studies attempt to find the connection between genetics and anxiety. One study used sets of identical and fraternal twins who were conditioned to generate a phobic response by pairing a picture with mild electrical shocks. When the fear response was learned, subjects had a fear reaction to the picture without the shocks. Researchers compared the responses between types of twins'. The identical twins who share the same genes had a similar response to the picture, while the fraternal twins' reactions varied. By studying the data, researchers concluded that anxiety has a genetic link.

As the technology for genetic testing advances, scientists will be able to continue to find genetic variants. Many researchers state that clearly heredity creates a propensity to develop anxiety disorders, but that no one gene will be the cause, and that environment and other factors, such as life experiences, will be as significant in determining who develops a disorder and who doesn't.

Biology

One of the factors in anxiety that is being studied is how your biological makeup affects your chances of developing an anxiety disorder. As you learned in Chapter 2, anxiety is a mind and body experience, and that the fear response is generated by the complex nervous system, which includes the brain, spinal cord, other organs, nerves, and chemicals. And common to all anxiety disorders is a state of intense arousal to either known or unknown stimuli. Many scientists believe that if there is a disturbance in the brain chemicals, then a malfunction will take place in your response and arousal to perceived danger. The glitch results in increased sensitivity and panicky responses to experiences, which you perceive as serious. For example, if you experience heart palpitations, you may interpret them as the beginning of a heart attack.

 Fact

Dr. Jerome Kagan of Harvard studied children with separation anxiety disorder (SAD) and found that children who were "behaviorally inhibited," or shy were more likely to develop SAD, which he attributed to biological, genetic, and environmental reasons. Kagan found that children with SAD had a common physiological trait, a high resting heart rate and, when stressed, their heart rate rose even higher. Parents of these children were also more likely to have an anxiety disorder.

The Amygdala

Other investigators looking into the biological causes of anxiety, using brain scans and other techniques, are studying the hippocampus and amygdala, both of which are involved in regulating emotions and storing memory. The amygdala, located in the limbic system, the seat of emotions, is thought to be the center of communications between the processes of incoming sensory information and the elements of the brain that read and understand the signals.

The workings of the amygdala are seen clearly in a phobic reaction. Let's say a child has a frightening experience with a large spider, and every time after that, when he sees a spider, or even a picture of a spider, he has a phobic reaction and screams and runs away. It's the amygdala that is involved in communicating to the brain, "A spider. Danger, danger!!" Even if the danger is only in a picture, remember the brain does not know the difference between real or perceived threat. The body will rev up the "fight or flight," and the child will flee to safety.

The Hippocampus

The hippocampus, involved in the functioning of the limbic system, processes dangerous or traumatic experiences and events. It also plays a role in storing information into memory. Through brain imaging, researchers studying posttraumatic stress disorder found that the hippocampus appears to be smaller in individuals who have experienced severe trauma, for example, being involved in military combat, or crime victims. This change in the hippocampus could account for the flashbacks and memory difficulties in people with PTSD. Ongoing research looking for the causes of and new treatments for obsessive-compulsive disorder include studying other parts of the brain; for example, the basal ganglia, which is found at the base of the brain and is involved in movement, cognition, and emotion.

Personality

What exactly is personality? It is defined as enduring characteristics, which include attitudes, beliefs, thoughts, habits, emotions, and behaviors that make you unique. Many theories exist about personality development, but exactly how the complex interplay of biological, psychological, and sociological factors makes us tick is still unknown, and an area of continued study.

In studying anxiety disorders, researchers found that people who develop them share many of the same characteristics in their personalities and labeled them "high anxiety personality types." Experts believe that having these qualities put an individual at a higher risk for developing an anxiety disorder. Some of these qualities include:

- *High degree of creativity and imagination*: Severe anxiety creates worry about what might happen in future situations. If you have this trait, you have a tendency to carry around vivid mental pictures of yourself in frightening situations.
- *Rigid thinking*: Seeing the world in terms of black-and-white thinking, with either/or an inflexible right or wrong attitude. This way of thinking leaves no room for the gray areas of life. The person may be uptight, tense, and unforgiving of himself and others.
- *Extreme need for acceptance*: Those with low self-esteem need approval from others to feel worthwhile. They are likely to be sensitive to criticism and will do anything for others to avoid rejection. These people also have a tendency to be taken advantage of.
- *Perfectionism*: This trait includes: having unrealistic goals that can never be achieved, thus setting yourself up for failure; focusing on minor mistakes or flaws instead of seeing the positive; chronic worry that you said or did the wrong thing; and comparing yourself negatively to others.
- *Need to be in control*: Some need to direct and manage life to keep anxious feelings from arising and feel distressed when the unpredictable occurs. These people often appear calm but suffer from inner turmoil, worrying about what might happen, and struggling to control themselves, others, circumstances, and events.

Other high anxiety traits are stifling or burying your feelings because you are afraid that you will either lose control or cause someone to be angry at you. You ignore physical signs of stress, such as feeling depleted, or being in pain, and do not get the rest and relaxation you need.

Having the personality traits listed here is not a sure sign that you will develop an anxiety disorder. In fact, all of us have some of these characteristics, which can be positive in some situations. For example, being detailed oriented, and a hard worker who puts in long hours does not make you a perfectionist. Or wanting to know the outcome of something important does not mean you are a control freak. It's a matter of degree, severity, and how your life is being affected that determines whether these qualities are working for or against you.

Essential

Personality disorders differ from personality traits. They are defined as ingrained, inflexible widespread patterns of behavior that deviate from cultural norms and cause severe distress and impairment in the individual's personal and occupational life. Examples of personality disorders are obsessive-compulsive personality disorder, dependent personality disorder, and borderline personality disorder.

Childhood Factors

The environment plays a major role in who will and who will not develop anxiety disorders. Researchers have long studied the connection between genetics and the innate qualities of temperament and how childhood experiences and parenting style are a predictor of what children are at risk for developing anxiety disorders sometime in their lives. Studies show that babies born with tendencies to be overexcited or fearful in some situations may not develop anxiety disorders if they are parented in a certain way. Research that has continued for decades indicates that two types of parenting style correlate with a higher risk of anxiety disorders in their children.

Overprotective Parenting Style

Overprotective parents try to shield their children from stressful situations, instead of letting them work out life's day to day problems. In his studies, Dr. Jerome Kagan found that 40 percent of infants with reactive temperaments whose parents were overprotective were more fearful and showed signs of distress by the age of two when exposed to strange places, events, and people, than those with parents who had an authoritative parenting style.

Rejecting or Neglectful Parenting Style

The other parenting styles are the rejecting or neglectful parent, who is aloof and lacks emotional warmth. Some studies found that mothers of children who were anxious were more controlling and negative in their interactions with their children. Neglectful parents may make the child feel lonely, unaccepted, and unprotected. Rejecting parents are usually highly critical and children from these parenting situations feel unwanted and unloved. Both situations lead to children growing up with low self-esteem and poor life coping skills.

Childhood Parental Experiences Linked to Anxiety Disorders

Parenting styles, events, and experiences all have a profound effect on a child developing an anxiety disorder at some point in their life. Parents who are substance abusers and are unstable, violent, and neglectful commonly have children who grow up being tense and afraid along with developing low self-esteem. Children who experience physical, sexual, and emotional violence, cruelty, and emotional abandonment become wounded adults who have a hard time functioning in the world and have an extremely high risk for anxiety disorders, as well as substance abuse, and other mental and physical disorders. Separation or loss of a parent through death, divorce, or emotional abandonment can lead to separation anxiety disorder and open the child up to other anxiety disorders later in his or her life.

Children who have anxious parents are most likely genetically loaded for anxiety and learn from their parents that going out into the world causes anxious feelings. Parents who are critical or are rigid and perfectionists have children with low self-esteem, who do not feel capable, and grow into tense and anxious adults. Parents who do not allow for an expression of feelings often have children who cut themselves off emotionally and, over time, this "suppression" leads to the inability to handle emotions. Not knowing how to express your feelings and emotions in a healthy way creates tension, anxiety, and depression. Children with alcoholic parents may grow up with an excessive need to control life's situations, or others who suffered abuse may have an extreme need for approval.

 Fact

One study examined parents with social phobia, other mental disorders, and parenting style for the risk of social phobia in their children. The results showed that there was a strong correlation between parents with social phobia, depression, alcohol use, and overprotective and rejecting parenting styles and social phobia in their children.

Anxiety Theories

Theories attempt to explain certain facts or phenomena. Psychological theories try to understand and explain the workings of the mind, and detail a method for treating mental disorders. Psychological theories on the development of anxiety disorders and how to treat them are numerous and go back to the beginning of civilization. There are numerous theories and therapies it is important to know about.

Psychodynamic Theories

Psychoanalytic theory, founded by Sigmund Freud, poses that anxiety originates in infancy and childhood stemming from unconscious conflicts of sexual feelings toward parents or other adults. The modern psychodynamic theories also look at unresolved childhood issues that manifest as emotional symptoms. As an example, childhood abuse can lead to the development of an anxiety disorder such as posttraumatic stress disorder. Or phobias are believed to be caused by "displacement," where a person unconsciously switches their feelings from an anxiety producing person or object, to one that is benign. For most psychodynamic theories, anxiety is caused by unresolved relationships and anger. These theories are difficult to do scientific studies on because emotions, unconscious conflicts, and drives are not tangible, and it is difficult to find empirical evidence, but new technology (scans, imaging) is researching the effects of psychotherapy on the brain.

Learning Theories

From the time we were born, we have been learning but are not always aware of doing so. We know as children that our parents taught us how to dress ourselves, eat by ourselves, etc. Less obvious is that we also learned by watching our parents, called modeling, and learned attitudes, habits, and ways of thinking. If our parents were tense and anxious, had anxiety disorders, were afraid of new things and going out in the world, they heavily influenced us, and there's a good chance we learned to be afraid and anxious too.

Learning-behavioral theories have been studied by researchers extensively as a cause for anxiety disorders. One of the leaders in the field, Albert Bandura, studied observational learning, beginning in the 1960s. In one study, Bandura had children watch a film where an adult aggressively hit and kicked a large doll. In one film, some of the children saw the adult being rewarded for the attack; in another, the adult was punished, in the last film, no reward or punishment was forthcoming. When the children were put in the room with the doll, those who saw the adult rewarded for aggression were the most aggressive. Bandura demonstrated that we do learn through modeling, but how children are reinforced seems to determine if the behavior will be copied.

Classical and Operant Conditioning

Other learning theories include Pavlov's classical conditioning (associative learning) where, for example, a scary or frightening thing is paired with something safe, and the person begins to identify the safe thing with the scary thing. Let's say a child, who is in an automobile accident and traumatized, will probably associate riding in a car with fear, when before the accident, he thought riding in the car was fun.

Operant conditioning, based on B. F. Skinners's research, is learning that occurs due to the results of the person's behavior, and the probability that behavior will be repeated. For example, you begin having panic attacks in malls. Soon you are anticipating having a panic attack on the way to the mall, and your anxiety increases. When you avoid the mall, your anxiety decreases and you don't have an anxiety attack. So, you begin avoiding malls all together. You learned that "avoidance behavior" makes you feel better, so there is a good chance you will repeat it.

L Essential

Classical and operant ways of learning are used in treatment. In classical, counterconditioning is used to reverse the undesirable effects of the prior conditioning—for example, giving the phobic child a special treat while he's taking a car ride. In operant learning, the reinforcer might be the panicky person feeling more confident when he has faced his fears and gone into a mall, or buying something special for himself at the mall.

Mental Conditions

Individuals diagnosed with mental disorders other than anxiety disorders may also experience severe anxiety. It is important for mental health practitioners to determine if the anxiety is a symptom of the condition, or is a co-morbid condition that needs to be treated separately. For example, people diagnosed with major depression often experience anxiety, too, or have an anxiety disorder like panic disorder. There are many conditions that have anxiety as a major component, and following are the most common ones.

Mental Disorders with a Component of Anxiety

Attention-deficit/hyperactivity disorder is a pattern of inattention, hyperactivity, and impulsivity that causes difficulty in daily functioning for children and adults. Substance-related disorders often develop because self-medicating makes it easier to cope with emotions and life circumstances. Schizophrenia is a psychotic disorder where the person loses touch with reality, leading to the inability to function in the world. People with depressive disorders that include major depressive disorder, dysthymic disorder, or bipolar disorders often have anxiety, obsessions, and phobias. Somatoform disorders include pain disorder, and hypochondriasis. Eating disorders, anorexia nervosa and bulimia nervosa are both associated with severe anxiety. Adjustment disorder with anxiety/with mixed anxiety and depressed mood are significant emotional responses to recognizable psychosocial stressors, for example, divorce, or losing one's job. And people with personality disorders are at a very high risk for anxiety, especially in dependent, borderline, and obsessive-compulsive personality disorders.

Question

What is sleep terror disorder?

Sleep terror disorder, also referred to as "night terrors," is repeated awakening due to frightening dreams, with screaming, yelling, crying, rising from the bed, punching, hitting, and slapping as if to fight off the terror. The person cannot remember the dream, or the incident. Sleep terrors cause major disruption in the person's ability to function in daily life. This condition is often found in people with posttraumatic stress disorder.

That list is only the most common disorders linked with anxiety. Of the 300-plus disorders listed in the DSM-IV, many more may have an accompanying anxiety component, making it difficult to determine an accurate diagnosis and then plan the most effective treatment.

Medications, Stimulants, and Illegal Drugs

Medications, stimulants, and illegal drugs all have the potential to create feelings of anxiety, mood swings, and changes in behavior. Many drugs can cause anxiety disorders to develop. These substances, which also include prescribed and over-the-counter medicines, may interact badly with medications you are already taking, or trigger anxiety because of their chemical properties. Illegal drugs such as marijuana have shown to have a strong link to the development of panic disorder. These substances include:

- Medications for cardiac and high blood pressure
- Drugs that treat ulcers
- Steroids
- Amphetamines, appetite suppressants
- Sleeping pills
- Antihistamines, cold remedies

Nicotine, caffeine, and alcohol are closely associated with causing anxiety disorders either in the use of, or during withdrawal. Recreational drugs that include cocaine, heroine, cannabis (marijuana), ecstasy, etc., are culprits in many of the cases of substance-induced anxiety disorder. Sometimes the anxiety begins with abuse of the substance but may not occur until the person tries to withdraw from the drug. Remember to always report all the medications and substances that you are taking to your doctor.

Essential

Prednisone, an anti-inflammatory used for diseases such as arthritis may cause mood changes in short term use, such as anxiety, depression, and feelings of being "hyper." Studies show that very high doses of prednisone, 40 mg. or more, taken on a daily basis may cause "steroid psychosis." Symptoms include anxiety, pressured speech, auditory and visual hallucinations, and memory impairment.

Significant Life Events

The importance of life events on how you feel and behave cannot be underestimated. All around us are the stressors that impact us: loss, death, change. How the stressful event is perceived conditions how we will cope with it. Stress builds up over time, accumulated by the myriad of events that we are part of. Significant life events that require a major life transition can be exceedingly stressful: changing jobs, losing jobs, leaving a significant relationship, moving, the death of a loved one are extremely difficult to cope with. While dealing with one or two events a year is doable, accumulated events that stretch over many years with added ones tacked on as time passes can lead to chronic stress and exhaustion. Significant life events include:

- Children leaving home
- Getting married
- Death of a parent
- Pregnancy
- Buying a house

It is known that stress can influence your risk of developing high blood pressure, ulcers, and headaches. Recent research reveals that accumulation of stress, banked over time, can impact the brain and cause the development of anxiety disorder and other mental conditions. Additionally, other factors that add to your risk of anxiety are heredity, which may play a large role in your responses, and childhood experience.

Traumatic Experiences

Trauma is a distinct experience that creates physical and emotional distress that may lead to posttraumatic stress disorder and other serious mental and physical conditions. The main characteristic of a traumatic experience is that the person is helpless to stop the event or circumstance from occurring. Traumatic events include a physical attack on your person, attacks on your city or country, serious illness, sexual harassment/rape, and military combat.

Fact

Not everyone who experiences a traumatic event develops an anxiety disorder. There are many factors that influence who develops anxiety and an anxiety disorder, and who doesn't. These include severity and duration of the trauma, the individual's ability to handle the situation, what support for the person is available, and his age.

The complexity of anxiety and anxiety disorders creates physical, emotional, and mental distress, and anxiety disorders are not easily remedied. Because there is no known single cause and anxiety is a unique human experience, finding an effective treatment can be difficult and frustrating. Ongoing research into conventional and alternative treatments continues to find new medications and therapies.

CHAPTER 11

Characteristics Associated with Anxiety

People with anxiety disorders are thought to have what is called a "high anxiety personality." This personality type is associated with certain characteristics that are believed to be part of the reason that anxiety develops. Not all people who have anxiety will have all of these traits, but it is likely one or more will exist. This chapter focuses on these characteristics and how they manifest themselves in a person's life.

Self-Esteem and Self-Worth

The development of a positive self-image is very important to your overall happiness. If you carry a positive view of yourself it is more likely that you are an independent adult who can take care of yourself in life. You are more apt to want to try new things. You can go after your dreams and work to accomplish your goals. Failure and disappointment are to be learned from and you do not get emotionally devastated when these things occur. High self-worth means you are likely to be able to handle both your positive and negative emotions. You can give your care and support to others more easily and freely.

Low Self-Esteem

Low self-esteem and low self-worth are based on the negative views you have of yourself. If you have low self-esteem, you may experience some or all of the following.

- Feel afraid to try new things
- Feel that you do not have the capacity to accomplish anything

- Blame others for your disappointments and failures
- Always compare yourself to others
- Feel that no one cares about you, or is willing to support you

Positive self-esteem is not something you wake up with one day. It is an aspect of your "self" that began in childhood and impacts your life at every age. If you think that you have low self-esteem, think about how long you have felt this way. Many people with this condition have had low self-esteem for as long as they can remember. However, low self-worth is not set in stone—with hard work you can convert negative to positive.

Anxious/Critical Parents

One aspect of developing good self-esteem is what you have learned from your parents or guardians. If your parents had feelings of positive self-worth, then it would be likely that you would too. But if they were not confident and critical most of the time, then they may have been unhappy and had trouble coping with life's stressors. Perhaps you were not allowed to make decisions, did not learn how to express your emotions in a healthy way, or weren't supported or nurtured—these all lead to low self-esteem, which increases your risk for anxiety.

Parental/Guardian Loss

If as a child or adolescent you experienced the death of a parent, were a child of divorce, or were separated from parents or guardians for a long time, you have suffered a great loss, or in some cases, a trauma. Young children have a difficult time making sense of the loss but often feel that their life has become unstable. Older children and adolescents understand cognitively what has occurred but often experience feelings of being abandoned and rejected by the parent who is no longer there. They also report feeling unsure and unstable about what the affects of the loss of their life will be, for example, having to move away from school and friends after a divorce. If children are not helped by adults to cope with the loss and their grief, and not made to feel stable, they often develop low self-worth and are at risk to develop emotional disorders.

Child Abuse

If you have suffered from physical or verbal abuse as a child, it is likely that you have developed a low regard for yourself. Children take verbal abuse as literal, "gospel," and believe that they are bad, stupid, ugly, unworthy, or whatever else a parent, guardian, teacher, or other adult tells them. Children who are physically or sexually abused have been traumatized. They live in fear, never knowing when their reactions will bring on yelling, hitting, or other abusive actions. Children and adolescents who were abused often present posttraumatic stress disorder. Building positive self-regard in children comes out of nurturing and love, not abuse and fear.

Question

What is negative self-talk?
This term describes the things you tell yourself to bring yourself down. One way to begin to counter negative self-talk is by consciously switching to positive affirmations. For example, "I'll never get a promotion," can be changed to, "I will work harder and become more engaged in my work." Affirmations should be personal and meaningful.

Addiction

Children of parents/guardians who are addicted to alcohol, drugs, sex, spending money, or work have a high risk of growing up with a sense of low self-worth. It is estimated that in the United States, 20 million children come from households whose parents are addicted to drugs and alcohol. These families are often unstable and chaotic and are a cause of trauma. Adults who are addicted may neglect and abuse their children. Children often have to "parent" their parents and don't get their own needs met. Children from addictive households do not usually form strong emotional bonds with parents, have low self-worth, and are at high risk for developing anxiety, depression, and self-defeating and self-destructive behaviors.

How Does Self-Esteem Relate to Anxiety?

Think of anxiety as a good thing, as much a part of your life as eating or sleeping. Anxiety can be a beneficial spur keeping you on your toes, readying you to deal with the challenges you face. By the same token, anxiety or fear that overwhelms and interferes with daily living can paralyze you. If you have good self-esteem, you accept yourself and roll with the punches. If you have low self-esteem, you carry the burden of not knowing who you are and are anxious and are likely to be stymied in fulfilling your life goals. These feelings can provoke terrible anxiety that is hard to control. The good thing about low self-esteem is the fact that it can be changed. You can build your confidence, and with it comes feeling good about yourself, and high self-worth.

Perfectionism

Perfectionism has both positive and negative features. It drives you to do good work, to challenge yourself, and to move toward goals. But one of the downsides of perfectionism is that you are unable to feel the satisfaction of a job well done.

If you are a perfectionist, you never think things are done exactly right or good enough. You are dissatisfied with yourself and others. You set goals that are unachievable and set yourself up for failure. In a positive direction, perfectionism provides the drive, which can lead to specific achievement. Having high standards to do the best job you can, or setting high goals for yourself is important for building confidence and self-worth. If you are a perfectionist, you relentlessly exert yourself toward unreasonable goals that cannot be met, and then measure your self-worth by your failure to accomplish them.

Characteristics of Perfectionism

If you are a perfectionist, you have a number of characteristics that are driving you to seek the impossible—pure perfection. Perfectionism is an internal learned coping mechanism, but it can be unlearned. The following are some of the characteristics of perfectionism:

- Fear of making mistakes
- Fear of failure
- Fear of being rejected and disliked
- High level of anxiety
- Black and white thinking
- Use of words like "never," "should," and "always"

Fact

Perfectionism exacts a great toll from individuals who think that only through perfection will they be able to gain the fulfillment, success, love, and acceptance of others. Usually, the opposite occurs. Perfectionists may accomplish something but, invariably, their methods will deny them the precise love and acceptance they badly wish to acquire, which leaves them always feeling dissatisfied.

As a perfectionist, you may be very driven to succeed to make up for feeling badly about yourself but are at a high risk for being highly stressed and suffering from fatigue and chronic burnout.

Accepting an Imperfect World

If you can learn to accept that there's no perfect way to feel, no perfect way to do something, you won't get bogged down pressuring yourself to do things precisely perfect. That approach will only make you miserable, and your performance will likely suffer if you try to live up to unrealistic expectations. Your anxiety will be high, if that's how much pressure you put on yourself. Learning to let go of your perfectionism is hard to do but the benefits are worth the effort.

One of the characteristics of being a perfectionist is the difficulty in forming close relationships. If you are hard on yourself, you may be unforgiving of others too. But as you let go of being a perfectionist, you'll find that people will react differently to you. They will want to work with you and spend time with you now that you are not so tense and uptight.

L Essential

Once you've determined that there's no perfect way to feel, or to do something, people's opinions won't drive you into a fetal position. They don't determine how you feel about yourself, or whether you're a worthy person—you do. You'll find that it's a great relief to say things to yourself like, "I don't know."

Repressed Emotions

In our culture anger and other feelings are often inadequately expressed. Strong feelings and emotions are usually avoided, or dealt with superficially, because they are so uncomfortable to accept and face. When we bury emotions like anger it is in our unconscious mind. It is out of the here and now, but it is not erased and will cause problems in the form of symptoms such as anxiety and depression. This is also true for embarrassing or frightening feelings you don't want to have to deal with. Such emotions, as violent feelings of rage, fear of rejection, or of being unloved, feel too scary or painful. But if these feelings are not expressed in appropriate and healthy ways, then inner tension builds and you put yourself at risk for developing emotional and psychosomatic symptoms. These include: extreme tension and anxiety, ulcers and other stomach problems, back pain, hypertension, chronic pain and body aches, hives, and skin rashes.

Repressed anger may also be directed at the self, that is, anger turned inward. If you turn your emotions on to yourself, you may experience depression to go along with your anxiety. Or maybe you spend a lot of your time concentrating on somatic problems, such as migraines, chronic fatigue, having difficulty remembering things, etc. If this is what is happening to you, you may be avoiding dealing with unexpressed emotions.

Alert

Keeping your feelings bottled up can cause potentially destructive mental and physical stress. In addition, your repressed feelings can burst out at inappropriate occasions, for example, outbursts of anger that is far in excess of what is warranted in the situation, making you feel remorseful and guilty. This only leads to a cycle of more anxiety and other emotional problems.

Expressing Your Emotions

If you believe that you are repressing your emotions and that they are making you anxious and sick, you can do a number of things to help yourself:

- Speak to a therapist or counselor to uncover why you feel the way you do. Becoming aware of unconscious feelings and accepting them as natural to the human condition will help you feel emotionally lighter and physically healthier. You also want to learn how to cope with strong emotions in an appropriate manner.
- Since anxiety is a mind-body experience, become involved with an exercise program that meets your physical needs. Physical exercise helps to lessen the grip of anxiety on your mind and will relieve stress and tension. Even regularly taking a slow walk has been shown to relieve emotional barriers.

- Learn how to relax and open yourself to the things around you that might bring you happiness or contentment. Taking a moment to enjoy life may relieve your emotional pressure cooker for a little while and lift your mood.

If you are interested in finding out what is bothering you, or seeking relief from anxiety in some of the other ways listed, be sure to have a discussion with your family physician, especially if you want to start an exercise program. Bringing your emotions to the surface, and facing them is not easy, and may be uncomfortable to do, but the benefits will be a more relaxed and healthier you.

Need for Approval

People with healthy self-esteem, who are not chronic worriers, or have anxiety, are able to put into perspective any disapproval or criticism they may experience. If you feel like this, then being criticized will not destroy your inner security. Though most people like to have approval from others, a person with high self-regard is not "dependent" on the approval or disapproval of others. On the other hand, if you have low self-esteem, and lack that sense of inner security, you may need the approval of others, to feel good about yourself. This excessive need has been termed "approval addiction," and the basis for it is an irrational belief that others determine your worth.

People who have an extreme need for approval don't make waves; avoid conflict because someone may disapprove of them; work hard to keep relationships going no matter what the cost; will do anything to avoid conflict, even if it means agreeing to things they don't like; try to meet everyone else's needs except their own for fear of being rejected; agonize over the possible reactions to a decision they want to make; believe that nothing they do will bring enough approval; are easily defeated or quit if things don't go their way.

Approval seekers usually have very high anxiety and experience severe body tension. Stress levels are up most of the time due to chronic worrying about past interactions, and if they have done and said the "right" things. At the same time, it is common for people who need approval to almost always be concerned about what might occur in the future. If you have these traits, you might feel like you are in a "no win" situation, and that will create chronic stress and anxiety.

 Fact

> People who seek excessive approval have low self-esteem and feelings of diminished worth. Approval seekers are dependent on the validity of others and are driven to seek approval in any way. Sometimes they take their role models from unreal characters and situations on TV and the movies.

If you have a need to seek approval, you may find yourself at the mercy of the very people from whom you want a response. It is easy to be used or even abused by others if you need excessive approval. Still others may be turned off by the need for approval from them and will never give it, or discontinue the relationship with you.

Rigid Thinking

If you experience chronic anxiety, it is likely that one of your characteristics is rigid thinking. Rigid thinking is to think in "either-or" terms, and to want clear-cut, black and white answers. If you think in this way, then the "gray areas" of life are uncomfortable for you. Other characteristics include:

- Things are either "right" or "wrong," "good" or "bad"
- Often have an "exact" way of doing things with no variations
- Have a tendency to be pessimistic
- Are unable to change
- Are very hard on yourself

If you are a rigid thinker you may have difficulty with relationships because the ability to see someone else's point of view is absent. To have a good relationship you must compromise, have a give and take, which shows care and respect for others. If you are a rigid thinker you may have a hard time bending to make room for another person.

Essential

If you have rigid thinking, you may suffer from various psychological symptoms, among them are obsessive thinking and acting out compulsively. You may have a distorted view of yourself, for example, believing you are weak of character and can't change if you fail at something, or believing the same of others if they fail or disappoint you.

Tendency to Ignore Signs of Stress

The tendency to ignore physical and psychological signs of stress revolves around your anxiety or preoccupation with worry about your problems. Ignoring the stress is self-serving: if you ignore it, if it isn't there, then it won't have to be faced, nor will it require any response on your part. If you are generally "elsewhere" these days, out of touch with your body and yourself, you can ignore an entire range of symptoms that are warning signs that something is wrong. You could be heading for a fall, and ignoring all the signs until it's too late. Consider these tendencies:

- You deny you're experiencing stress and anxiety.
- You ignore physical symptoms of stress. For example, having high blood pressure.
- You avoid seeking help.
- You use nicotine, caffeine, or other drugs to self-medicate.
- You do not take time to rest and relax.

- You cannot manage your time well and have a hard time balancing work, family time, and leisure.

Before things get really out of hand, take time to see the reality of the whole picture. Then rather than deal with something so large and overwhelming, break it into doable parts and deal with each one, one at a time. There's much you can change on your own. Some things you will be better off getting help for. And each problem you tackle is another success, lessening anxiety and tension, building your confidence, and making your life more enjoyable.

Desire for Control

You have an extreme need to be in control because you don't want to have a moment's anxiety over anything. To be in control, you think, makes you feel better. If you need to be in control all the time you do it really to control your emotions, to keep them buried. The need to control means you do not like change of any kind, even if what is happening is uncomfortable or harmful to you. Change creates the unknown, and equals loss of control. You can't control what might happen in the future. You can't control other people, and trying to do so will ruin relationships, and keep people away from you. The only person you can learn to control is yourself.

Alert

Trying to keep total control over yourself, your environment, others, situations, and circumstances will only increase your tension, stress, and anxiety. The excessive need for control is "white knuckling" your way through life. You never reach that state of relaxation and ease where you can let go and just "be," because you live in a state of chronic worry about losing control.

Learning to Let Go

The only way to let go of control is to learn to take life as it comes. You need to learn to accept what you cannot change. Your life (everyone's life, in fact) is influenced by events over which we have no control. To loosen your grip on control, practice living in the present, learn to taste the unique experience of each new moment, strive to see and appreciate the beauty of the world around you, and recognize the limitations of life and try to accept them.

If you have high levels of anxiety, you may want to examine yourself for characteristics of the need for excessive control. Become aware of what happens to your body and mind when you feel anxious and you start trying to control everything around you. Look at how your breath becomes shallow, feel how rigid your head, neck, and shoulders become. Do you feel off balance and awkward at these times? Trying to control everything around you will not work. When you can let go, you'll fear less, and live more.

Distorted Thinking

The core of distorted thinking is an irrational or senseless perception of yourself in your world. This distorted point of view affects your decision making and interactions with those around you. This form of thinking comes out even more so when you're overly stressed, tired, anxious, or ill. Distorted thinking leads to flawed assumptions and incorrect conclusions. If you have to contend with the inability to see alternate solutions to problems, or set realistic goals, or make good decisions, you may find that you suffer from anxiety and depression.

Distorted thinking is also called dichotomous thinking, or all-or-nothing thinking. This type of thinking is in absolutes, black or white, good or bad, right or wrong. These thoughts create a distorted view of the world, by trying to fit all the complexities of life and people into a simplistic view. Because life is not simple, or easy, and people are complex, if you have distorted thinking, you will set yourself up for anxiety and depression.

Characteristics of Distorted Thinking

Your mistakes and flaws or those of others are magnified, and if you happen to make a mistake, you label yourself as worthless. You have a negative view of the word, and exaggerate situations and events—one little mistake becomes a catastrophe. You devalue personal strengths, abilities, and achievements, in yourself and others. Here's an example of an event and the distorted thinking reaction to it:

A friend calls you to cancel a bowling date because of illness. You're very disappointed and think, "I wonder if she is mad at me? She doesn't think I'm good enough but can't tell me to my face. She'll probably never call me again to go bowling." If you think in a distorted way, you may take responsibility for a negative occurrence when there's no foundation for doing so, and imagine what people are thinking or feeling with little or no basis to support your thoughts. You magnify everything out of proportion and make yourself the focus of the event.

Distorted thinking can exacerbate during stressful anxious times, and you need to be aware that this is happening. Accept it, and begin to slowly change the way you think. Also try to recognize distorted thinking in other people, which will help you become more aware of your own distorted thoughts.

If you have an anxiety disorder, you may have recognized some of these characteristics in your own personalities. Try not to feel distressed or hopeless because of this. Each of these characteristics has a positive side as well as a negative side, and all people have bits and pieces of these traits in them. It is when these characteristics stand in the way of living that you have to take action. If you are anxious and distressed, it is recommended that you do some soul searching, either by yourself, with a trusted friend, or with a mental health practitioner, to see what characteristics you'll have to accept, which ones you want to change, and how to utilize the positive aspects of these personality characteristics.

Chapter 12

Conditions Linked to Chronic Anxiety

Stress and anxiety affect both mind and body, and if they become chronic, they can lead to other physical illnesses and emotional conditions. Researchers have been studying the connection between stress, anxiety, and physical ailments for decades, in hopes of finding preventative techniques. This chapter examines the diseases and conditions that may be caused by chronic anxiety and offers tips on how to detect the onset of a problem.

Where's the Connection?

Stress is the body's physical response to events and circumstances. Stress is both a positive and negative force and the characteristics of stress are the same whether you are being held up at gunpoint, or cashing in a jackpot lottery ticket. The stress response is the "fight or flight" reaction and includes the following changes:

- Blood pressure rises
- Stress hormones such as adrenaline are released into the bloodstream
- Heart rate becomes rapid
- Breathing becomes rapid and shallow
- Muscles tense
- Sweating occurs

Stress: A Part of Life

The occurrence of stressful situations is a natural part of life. At those times, your body revs itself up to meet the threat, and the sympathetic nervous system engages the "fight or flight" response, which produces symptoms of anxiety. When the stressor (whatever it is that is making demands on the body) is no longer present, the relaxation response kicks in so the body can renew its resources.

Sometimes, your response to stress is a normal adaptive reaction to what is happening. But maladaptive reactions to stress can occur that include poor coping skills, denial of stress on your body, unhealthy, destructive coping strategies, and the inability to handle your emotions. When you get overwhelmed about the stress in your life and it becomes chronic it may lead to any number of anxiety disorders, and physical ailments.

L. Essential

The link between chronic stress and disease has been studied extensively beginning in the 1950s, and by 1956 the term "stress" had become part of American speech. Thomas Holmes, a physician and researcher, studied the connection between stress and tuberculosis (TB). Holmes found that patients who experienced stressful situations, for example, divorce, or death of a spouse, were less likely to recover from the disease.

The Effects of Stress

People who are unable to adapt to stressful situations have a high risk of anxiety, depression, and physical illnesses. Stress affects us on many levels: emotionally, when we become depressed, anxious, hopeless, and lose our zest for living; socially, if we withdraw from family and friends and feel isolated; mentally, when we find it difficult to concentrate or make decisions and become uninterested in pursuing life goals.

Researchers have looked at what happens when the stress response is activated throughout the day, and the body's normal resting state does not occur. Their studies show that the recurrence of release of stress hormones, such as cortisol, produces hyperactivity in certain areas in the nervous system, namely the hypothalamus, pituitary, and adrenal glands. When the pituitary and adrenal glands release hormones, the hypothalamus, which controls the stress response, causes levels of cortisol to rise. Cortisol is the steroid hormone that helps us handle stressful situations. In recent studies, researchers learned that the brain also uses cortisol to suppress the immune system, and decrease inflammation in the body. This suppression of the immune system may be one major link between the body's decreased ability to ward off disease due to chronic stress.

When stress is unrelenting, it can cause major damage to every part of your body. Chronic stress can also occur when many little stressors accumulate over time, keeping the body in an almost constant state of arousal. Consider the following case example:

> Karen, who was in a verbally abusive marriage for fifteen years, was diagnosed with a pain disorder six years into the marriage. Right after her fifteenth wedding anniversary, she was diagnosed with breast cancer. When she went to see a mental health clinician, she acknowledged that her father, who was an alcoholic, was also verbally abusive, and that she felt very frightened and anxious throughout her life. Through counseling, she realized that she had a very high risk of developing a major disease because she had been living with chronic stress since she was a child.

Stress, and the anxiety it produces, can depress the body's immune and inflammatory systems making you more susceptible to viruses, colds, and other diseases, as well as exacerbating diseases such as cancer, multiple sclerosis, AIDS, and arthritis. The rapid breathing associated with the stress response can worsen the symptoms of asthma and other respiratory diseases. The list of stress-related diseases is long and some experts contend that stress plays a major role in the development of many diseases.

🖼 Fact

Studies show that increased stress response activity disrupts the balance in the body's normal functioning. When you are stressed, levels of serotonin, which is one of the major chemicals in the brain involved in regulating moods, decrease. Serotonin promotes feelings of being calm and relaxed, and sleepiness. That is why chronic stress can cause insomnia and disruption in daily living.

Cardiovascular Disease (CVD)

Cardiovascular diseases kills about one million Americans a year and is the leading cause of death for both men and women thirty-five years and older, and cuts across all racial and ethnic groups. One out of every four Americans has cardiovascular disease, that is almost 57 million people. CVD costs a staggering $274 billion each year, which includes health costs and lost productivity. As the population ages, the costs are expected to grow. There are a number of different cardiovascular diseases and conditions that cause dysfunction of the arteries and veins in the heart that supply oxygen to the heart, brain, and other crucial organs.

Cardiovascular Diseases and Conditions

The following is a list of cardiovascular diseases and conditions that can result from chronic stress:

- *Arteriosclerosis*: The narrowing and hardening of the arteries of the heart due to a buildup of plaque. Chest pains and angina pectoris may occur, leading to a major heart attack.
- *Hypertension (high blood pressure)*: Develops because of arteriosclerosis, a narrowing and hardening of the arteries. This buildup makes the heart work harder, eventually weakening the heart. If untreated, hypertension, which is called the "silent killer," may result in a heart attack or stroke.

- *Arrhythmia*: Is an abnormal heart rate caused by a disorder in the electrical impulses of the heart. Atrial fibrillation is when the heart beats at 300 to 500 times per minute. The most common cause of arrhythmia is arteriosclerosis.
- *Myocardial infarction (heart attack)*: A heart attack occurs when part of the heart muscle suddenly dies. If you survive the attack, you have an increased risk of having another within a few years.
- *Stroke*: Is damage to the brain caused when blood supply is disrupted, or blood leaks outside of blood vessel walls. Strokes cause impairment to the part of the brain that has been affected. Strokes are fatal in one third of cases.
- *Angina*: Is chest pain that ranges from mild to severe, due to a shortage of oxygen flowing to the heart muscle. It may occur when you are stressed and anxious, and when you are exerting yourself physically. Angina is dangerous; it is the precursor to a full-blown heart attack.

Alert

Smoking is a critical factor in your developing heart disease. Nicotine and other toxins in cigarettes damage blood vessels, increase the heart rate, and reduce the amount of oxygen to organs. Smoking also increases LDL cholesterol levels, which creates an increased risk of arteriosclerosis, and hypertension. Nicotine has been linked to increased anxiety and depression.

High cholesterol levels are an indicator of a high risk of heart disease, as is endocarditis, an infection of the heart. Other conditions that cause heart problems are valve disorders, liver problems, and autoimmune diseases, such as rheumatic fever and AIDS.

Causes of Developing CVD

According to studies, even the region you live in can be a factor in the development of heart disease, due to daily stressors, environmental pollution, and general lifestyle. Psychological stress, anxiety, and trauma are linked to cardiovascular diseases. Research has shown that people who have experienced trauma, such as combat or rape are more likely to develop heart disease, because high stress is linked to high blood pressure.

Other psychological factors include people who are chronically stressed and anxious, anger easily, and who exhibit rigid, perfectionist thinking. Scientists have studied the physiological processes of people prone to high levels of stress and anxiety and have determined that fat deposits, inflammation of arteries, and unstable plaques (that will block arteries) result from these emotional states.

Cancer

Cancers are diseases that cause uncontrolled growth and the spread of abnormal cells, and if the spread is not stopped, death can occur. There are more than 100 types of cancers, all with the same basic characteristic, that is, cancer cells have the ability to reproduce themselves. Some of the more common cancers are bladder cancer, brain cancer, breast cancer, liver cancer, melanomas-skin cancers, prostate cancer, and bone cancers.

How Does Cancer Progress?

Cancer can occur in every part of the body. For example, though melanoma is generally thought to affect only the skin, it can spread to orifices in the head, including the eyes. When tumors are cancerous they are called "malignant" because they can spread to healthy tissue. Cancers do this by dividing and destroying the part of the body they are in, then spreading, called metastases. Cancer spreads through the lymphatic system, the bloodstream, or by invading healthy tissue.

L. Essential

> The American Cancer Society strongly recommends a stress management program as a healthy way to handle life's stresses, and keep your immune system working for you. Besides eating right and exercising, tips include ways to stay calm and centered to keep the stress hormones, such as adrenaline, low through: deep breathing, meditation, imagery, and mindfulness.

Cancer and Stress

The connection between cancer and chronic stress and anxiety has been studied for years. Presently there is no definite scientific proof that emotions directly cause cancer. Some studies show that cancer patients who lower their stress levels increase their chance for survival. Other studies indicate that stress decreases the body's immune system, so that a person who is chronically stressed and anxious may be more open to certain kinds of cancer, since a healthy immune system is necessary to fight off the cancer causing agents we are exposed to daily. A number of studies showed significantly higher rates of breast cancer in women who had experienced traumatic events. Though many studies refute the link because of a lack of hard evidence, a number of scientists believe that though no hard evidence exists, the link is there, and how we respond to the stressors in our life makes the difference in how our body wards off disease.

Gastrointestinal Diseases

Gastrointestinal diseases affect the stomach and intestines, which is called the gastrointestinal tract. There are a variety of diseases, and they range from mild to severe and vary in symptoms. The main job of the stomach is to digest the foods we eat, by mixing the ingested food with enzymes and hydrochloric acid. When this process is disrupted, for example, a gastrointestinal disease will develop. These diseases include:

- Gastritis: inflammation of the gastric mucous membrane used in digestion
- Constipation or diarrhea
- Gastroesophageal reflux disease (GERD) or heartburn
- Irritable bowel syndrome (IBS): caused by sensitivity of nerves in the bowel
- Peptic ulcer: caused by a stomach-lining infection

As you've read in earlier chapters stress and anxiety wield power over the gastrointestinal tract, for stomach aches are one of the most common symptoms associated with stress and anxiety. All the functions associated with this tract, such as eating, digestion, and elimination are moderated by signals from nerve cells and hormones, which can be altered and disrupted due to anxiety.

Eating Disorders

The main feature of eating disorders is severe disturbances in eating patterns, which include behaviors such as starvation, binging, and purging. The National Institute of Mental Health estimates that between 5 to 10 million girls and women, and one million boys and men presently suffer from an eating disorder. One eating disorder is anorexia nervosa where the person refuses to eat enough food to maintain the minimal weight for age and height, is severely afraid of gaining weight, and has a significant distorted perception of the size and shape of their body. The person may either starve themselves (every year, more than 1,000 people in the United States die of starvation due to anorexia), or have periods of binging and purging. In bulimia nervosa the person uncontrollably binges and then purges through vomiting, misuse of laxatives, diuretics, fasting, and other means because they fear weight gain. The person's self-identity is based on their body shape and weight. Binge eating disorder is characterized by periods of uncontrollable binging, but not purging.

If you have an eating disorder you likely feel guilt and shame, and isolation. Experts believe that because of these feelings, many people with eating disorders, especially bulimia nervosa and binge eating disorder, are secretive about their problems, and many cases are unreported. And another group of people, it is believed, have sub-clinical eating disorders, for example, being abnormally obsessed with food or weight, but still fall within your "normal" weight range.

Researchers studying the connection between anxiety disorders and eating disorders found significant links between the two. And studies show that if both disorders exist, the symptoms of each disorder might worsen, and make treatment more difficult. For example, people who binge eat uncontrollably do so to relieve stress and anxiety. If the binging triggers fears of gaining weight and becoming fat, then the person might resort to either purging or restricting most food. But when the anxiety spikes again, a cycle of anxiety, binging, and purging or starvation will follow.

Alert

Since research studies have found a significant relationship between anxiety disorders and eating disorders, health care providers must be aware in initial evaluations to look for both disorders. If you have an eating disorder, or are preoccupied by your food intake, weight gain, and body shape, you may also be suffering from an anxiety disorder, and it is important to alert your health care provider to evaluate for both disorders.

Diabetes

Diabetes develops when the body does not produce enough insulin, which is a hormone that is needed to convert sugar and starch into energy. Type 1 diabetes is strictly an insulin production problem, but type 2 diabetes, includes failure to produce, and the body's inability to properly use insulin. It is estimated that 18.2 million Americans have diabetes, the majority being diagnosed with type 2. Of the estimated

18.2 million, 13 million have been formally diagnosed, but it is believed that more than 5 million people do not know they have the disease. Two other types of diabetes are: gestational diabetes: 4 percent of pregnant women develop diabetes only during their pregnancy; and prediabetes: a condition where book glucose levels are higher than normal, but do meet the criteria for a diagnosis of type 2 diabetes. It is estimated that 41 million people in the United States have prediabetes.

For decades researchers have been studying how stress and anxiety influences the course of diabetes. There is no proof that anxiety and other emotions cause diabetes, but studies show that stress and anxiety often cause big increases in blood glucose levels. Diabetics with panic disorder may experience either a jump or low levels of glucose during a panic attack, and it is important to carefully monitor glucose when stress and anxiety are high. Being properly diagnosed with a coexisting anxiety disorder is important so that proper treatment for the anxiety is begun as quickly as possible. Treating anxiety disorders is part of good management of diabetes.

Essential

Research on methods that will help keep blood glucose levels from fluctuating due to stress and anxiety include the use of relaxation techniques through yoga, meditation, and hypnotherapy. Recommendations also include getting involved in a moderate exercise program, which is a great way to handle the physiological effects of stress reactions. Remember to check with your doctor before starting an exercise program.

Pain

Chronic pain can develop in many areas of the body as a result of anxiety. Pain is distressing and debilitating and may significantly interfere with an individual's ability to function well in every aspect of their lives. Repeated doctor visits and expensive medical testing often fails to come up with a diagnosis, adding to the frustration and stress. Sometimes the chronic pain is caused by injuries to "soft tissue" that are slow to heal and difficult to diagnose. Experts think that the areas of the body that process pain can become dysfunctional, or slight damage to nerve cells may account for pain—but these are difficult to prove. Many painful disorders have no known origin, even with years of research looking for a cause.

Pain Sites in the Body

The following are places where you might experience pain in your body as a result of chronic anxiety:

- *Muscle contraction headaches*: These develop in the jaw and spread to either the sides of the head, forehead, back of head, and base of the skull.
- *Jaw pain*: Tension in the muscles around the temporomandibular joint (TMJ) causes headaches and pain in the mouth and teeth.
- *Neck and shoulder pain*: Most common place to store tension; may be caused by poor posture and anxious breathing patterns.
- *Lower back pain*: muscle tension in the back of upper legs will cause tension and pain in the lower back. Posture and anxious breathing patterns also play a role.

Conditions that have symptoms of body pain are fibromyalgia where aches and stiffness are all over your body, along with increased pain in "tender spots." Chronic fatigue syndrome features fatigue and body aches, and irritable bowel syndrome (IBS) symptoms are abdominal pain with diarrhea and constipation. Interstitial cystitis is bladder pain due to inflammation of bladder wall, and vulvodynia, which is pain in the external genitals of women.

Many sufferers of chronic pain believe that because their doctor cannot find the cause of their pain, their pain is all "mental," and not real. But pain, no matter the cause, whether a bump on the head, or due to extreme stress, is real. Doctors who specialize in pain disorders state that pain is a personal and unique experience, different for everyone.

Causes of Chronic Pain

Some of the possible explanations for chronic pain include experiencing stressful events in childhood, being more sensitive to pain due to sensitization of pain processing mechanisms in the body, disruption of your immune system, and being reinforced as a child that being sick leads to getting attention from parents.

Researchers have linked stress and anxiety to exacerbation and increased pain in people with chronic pain. Stress will trigger fibromyalgia flare-ups, and individuals with it often present with anxiety disorders and panic attacks. Extreme stress and anxiety has been linked to the development of chronic fatigue syndrome. And common treatments for pain conditions include stress management, relaxation techniques, and using calming breathing patterns.

Sexual Dysfunction

Sexual dysfunctions cover a wide range of conditions, which lead to problems that prevent people from experiencing satisfaction from sexual activity. Sexual dysfunctions are common, with 43 percent of women and 31 percent of men reporting sexual problems. Difficulties can be caused by physical or psychological problems. Male conditions include ejaculation disorders: premature, inhibited, and retrograde ejaculation that includes ejaculating before or right after penetration, ejaculation does not occur, and semen is forced into the bladder instead of out the penis. Erectile dysfunction (impotence) is the inability to achieve or maintain an erection for sexual intercourse.

Female conditions include female sexual arousal disorder, where a woman feels inhibited, does not get aroused, and may be repulsed when touched. Female orgasmic disorder where a woman is aroused but cannot reach orgasm, and vaginismus, involuntary spasm of the vagina making intercourse impossible. Disorders for both sexes include inhibited sexual desire, which is a decrease of loss of interest in sexual activity, and hypoactive sexual desire disorder, persistent repeated sex fantasies or desire for sex.

Sexual disorders are closely linked to stress and anxiety. Possible psychological causes include marriage or relationship problems, fears about sexual performance, having experienced a sexual trauma such as rape, and feeling guilty about having sex due to childhood upbringing, and finding your partner unattractive. Most sexual difficulties that occur because of stress and milder emotional disorders can be treated through counseling, sex education, and better communication with your partner. More severe emotional problems, such as having an anxiety disorder, may require psychotherapy and medication, though some medicines may exacerbate sexual problems.

Fact

Most people who seek help for sexual problems are between the late twenties and early thirties. But sexual dysfunction is also common in the aging population and usually related to the effects of aging. Sexual difficulties often cause distress and may create problems in a relationship. Men who experience sexual difficulties may feel shame and loss of control. Women may feel shame, isolation, and fear they are unattractive to their partner.

Allergies

It is estimated that more than 75 million Americans suffer from some kind of allergy. Allergies are the body's reactions to substances, such as foods and environmental matter like mold and spores. Allergies develop when the body does not recognize the substance, considers it foreign, and fights the substance by producing antibodies, or releasing chemicals called histamines. It is the histamines and antibodies that cause inflammation, which create the allergic reaction.

Allergy Symptoms

You may experience annoying seasonal allergies and get a stuffy, runny nose and watery eyes when spring arrives and plants throw off their pollen. But some allergic reactions are more severe and can cause distress, health problems, and death. There are hundreds of symptoms that result from allergens, including:

- Watery, itchy eyes, congested nose and sinuses, sneezing
- Respiratory problems
- Skin outbreaks
- Headaches
- Heart palpitations
- Fatigue
- Bloating/intestinal gas and pain
- Mood swings

Fact

Asthma is an allergic disorder where spasms of the air passages to the lungs cause shortness of breath and wheezing. Symptoms of an attack are frightening; tightness in the chest, problems in breathing and talking, and feelings of being suffocated are common. Diaphragmatic breathing has been used successfully in asthmatics to ease stress and anxiety and reduce the frequency of attacks.

Allergies fall into three types: natural environmental substances: mold, spores, pollen, grasses, flowers, dust, insects, animal hair; common food ones include: wheat, milk, eggs, corn, yeast, coffee, nuts, chocolate, shellfish; environmental and food chemicals include: food additives, pesticides, chemical sprays, hydrocarbons.

Psychological stress and anxiety have been linked to an increase in allergic reactions and symptoms. Research has shown that emotions play an important part in the severity of an individual's reaction to an allergen, and that learning to relax and reduce anxiety often relieves the symptoms of the allergic reaction.

Skin Disorders and Hair Loss

Skin is extremely vulnerable to stress and anxiety. Clinical trials prove that emotional stress and anxiety will harm your skin, and can lead to chronic skin disorders. Skin disorders are visible, sometimes lead to physical disabilities, scarring, etc., which can create additional psychological stress and negative feelings about appearance and self-worth. Common skin disorders include:

- *Acne*: occurs when pores in the skin become clogged causing pimples, and inflamed lesions
- *Psoriasis*: an inflammatory disease causing red, scaly plaques
- *Rosacea*: caused by excessive circulation, which creates a ruddy cast on the skin
- *Eczema/dermatitis*: inflamed and irritated skin disorders leading to dry, hot, itchy skin; sores; and bleeding

Essential

Some research into alternative treatments for skin diseases has focused on meditative techniques to promote healing. Patients with psoriasis were divided into two groups. Both groups were treated with conventional medicine, but one group also participated in meditation sessions. The group that meditated healed significantly faster.

Clinical trials of the link between skin disorders and stress and anxiety show that when an individual is stressed, the skin, whose job is as a barrier that keeps water inside of your body, malfunctions, causing dryness and leading to a host of skin conditions. The abnormality in the skin occurs when the person becomes anxious, and there is an increase in hormones, such as corticosteroids. These hormones have proven to be harmful to the skin. Acute stress, or long periods of stress and anxiety will do damage to your skin.

Hair loss is a devastating condition and has numerous causes. Emotional stress and anxiety has shown to cause hair loss. Case studies in the psychological literature report that patients have been treated for hair loss due to severe stress and anxiety. Physical illness and high fevers can cause hair loss. Chemicals and chemotherapy usually cause hair loss because they are toxic to the cells that reproduce hair. Physical traumas cause hair loss, as do changes in weight, pregnancy, and menopause. Some hair loss is attributed to hormones and genetics. Other hair loss conditions are caused by hormonal imbalances and autoimmune diseases. Hair loss conditions include: alopecia areata where hair loss may occur in areas of the scalp, the total scalp, or total body hair loss; male-pattern baldness where hair loss is seen on top of the head and sides of the head; female-pattern baldness where hair thins and loss is seen on of top of the head and sides of the scalp.

Hair loss affects 50 to 80 percent of Caucasian men, and numbers are smaller for other ethnic and racial groups. It is estimated that 20 to 40 percent of women in their late twenties and early forties develop hair loss, but because it is a devastating condition, it is a hidden condition. Though hair loss is psychologically difficult for both men and women, studies show that women have more emotional pain due to the loss. Cultural norms put more emphasis on physical appearance for women, so hair loss often leads to low self-esteem for women. Research has shown that women are more likely to suffer anxiety over hair loss and try to hide the loss with another style, consult a hair stylist, and work on other aspects of their appearance to take attention off of their hair loss.

The diseases and disorders described in this chapter are only some of the hundreds of illnesses and conditions that have been linked to the physiological reactions of the body when anxiety becomes chronic. As preventive "medicine," it is important to learn how to relax, rest, and de-stress to allow your mind and body to renew its resources. Other chapters in this book will give you information on techniques that can help you alleviate daily stress and anxiety.

CHAPTER 13

Psychological Testing

There are a number of tools that psychologists and mental health providers use to evaluate a person's personality and state of mind. Psychological testing is one of those methods. Psychological tests are also used for research purposes for a number of reasons, for example, to develop more effective treatment. This chapter covers psychological testing, its validity in diagnosis, and some of the specific tests that deal with anxiety.

What Is Psychological Testing?

Psychological testing (psychometrics), also called psychological assessment, is one of the ways that researchers or mental health practitioners measure and evaluate human behavior and abilities. The tests are standardized. Psychological tests are divided into a number of classifications: intelligence tests, achievement and aptitude tests, occupational tests, neuropsychological tests, and personality tests. Some tests measure for specific clinical criteria, for example, there are many tests whose goal is to find out information about panic disorder and agoraphobia.

If you have gone through the school system in the United States, then you have probably taken psychological tests, most likely IQ and aptitude tests. Psychological tests are produced and copyrighted by various test publishers, and only those professionals trained in psychological assessment are allowed to administer tests. Testing has its limitations because of the following: psychological tests have to be tested for validity and reliability for them to be able to measure what they were intended for; critics also site bias on the part of the evaluator. And experts point out that the human mind is just too complex to assess and evaluate with standard measures.

Some common tests include:

- *Intelligence tests:* These are standardized measures used to evaluate your cognitive function and intellectual competence usually for school and work. They are given to adults and children and its numerous subtests evaluate areas of intelligence like verbal and math skills, and spatial dexterity. IQ "norm" is 100.
- *Achievement and aptitude tests:* Achievement tests measure how much you know about a specific subject and are the most common tests used in schools. Your weekly spelling test, and the Scholastic Achievement Test (SAT), are examples. Aptitude tests measure your talents and interests.
- *Personality tests:* Personality tests try to uncover your personality type and are used in clinical settings to aid in diagnosis and in research labs. Personality tests measure aspects of your personality, such as self-esteem, how you cope under stress, and personality disorders.
- *Neuropsychological tests:* Neuropsychological tests measure your thinking ability, which includes how you speak, your logic and judgments, etc. Neuropsychological testing is often used to determine cognitive functioning due to disease, for example, dementia or brain injury.
- *Clinical tests for specific disorders:* These are used by clinicians to measure the degree of specific symptoms such as anxiety, panic attacks, agoraphobia, depression, and suicidal thoughts as part of a comprehensive evaluation. Many of these tests are self-administered.
- *Occupational tests:* The goal of occupational tests is to pair your talents and interests to certain jobs or professions. Your answers are scored and evaluated against the kinds of interests common to people who work in certain jobs. For example, if a large percentage of your interests match the interests of most lawyers, that might be the career choice for you.

L. Essential

> If you are going to be tested for anxiety, your health care clinician will still need to do an evaluation interview to find out about your family and background, attitudes about life, your symptoms, how you cope with anxiety and experience the world around you, and if you have other existing conditions or disorders.

Objective Personality Tests

Personality is defined as all of the attributes, such as qualities, characteristics, traits, and habits that make you a unique individual. Personality tests are used in a variety of settings to determine what these attributes are. Some of the tests are created with objective questions, such as the Minnesota Multiphasic Personality Inventory (MMPI), others like the Rorschach inkblot test are subjective and open to the interpretation of the evaluator's theory base. The MMPI is the most often utilized clinical test. It is used in legal trials to provide personality information on defendants, in custody cases, by psychologists, and in work related settings. The MMPI originated with a psychologist and a psychiatrist (Hathaway and McKinley) at the University of Minnesota in the late 1930s, with the object of speeding up diagnosis and treatment. In the beginning it was intended for use with an adult population but was expanded to include teenagers. The developers of MMPI wanted to differentiate what they called "pure" groups with psychiatric disorders. They did this by establishing ten clinical scales, three validity scales, and many supplementary scales:

- *Scale 1*: hypochondriasis scale
- *Scale 2*: depression
- *Scale 3*: hysteria
- *Scale 4*: psychopathic deviate scale
- *Scale 5*: masculinity-femininity

- *Scale 6*: paranoia
- *Scale 7*: psychasthenia scale
- *Scale 8*: schizophrenia scale
- *Scale 9*: hypomania scale
- *Scale 0*: social introversion

Researchers discovered that people often scored high on more than one scale at the same time and that evaluations using two or more scales tended to be more precise. The results of the MMPI are called a personality "profile."

Essential

The MMPI can be faked because of the obviousness of some of the items. Although the three validity scales can help the psychologist identify abnormal responses that might suggest faking, clients can angle their answers to give a favorable or unfavorable impression.

It is hard to regularly prejudice the MMPI because of the clarity and intricacy of the questions. Like all tests the MMPI has best results when it is interpreted with biographical data and other information about the client. The psychologist applying and interpreting the MMPI must be aware of all related and pertinent elements, including gender, age, education, religion, and other information that will make the interpretation valid.

The world's most widely used personality inventory, the MBTI® or Myers-Briggs Type Indicator was developed around the ideas and theories of Carl Jung. Briggs and Myers extended Jung's model with the initial development of the MBTI. They put Jung's concepts of personality types: sensing perception, intuition perception, thinking judgments, and feeling judgments into language easily understood by the average person. The MBTI is licensed in about twenty foreign languages and has been specially designed to be valid in other languages and cultures. Adaptations of the Myers-Briggs appear on many Web sites.

Subjective Personality Tests

A number of the specific tests used in psychodynamic assessment that are based on the person's interpretations of pictures, inkblots, etc., are called projective tests. These tests came out of Freudian and Neo-Freudian theories and are open to interpretation based on the therapist or evaluator's psychological theories. The Rorschach ink-blot test is a test used to analyze personality. The person taking the test tells the therapist what he or she sees in a series of ten bilateral symmetrical inkblot designs, and then the therapist interprets the information and discusses it with the client. Years of research has gone into standardizing the inkblot interpretations, and while the Rorschach test is the most accepted projective technique, objective tests such as the MMPI are more commonly used

 Fact

> The House-Tree-Person test (H-T-P) has no specific testing materials and cannot be standardized. In this test, the person is asked to draw a picture of a house, tree, and person, which is interpreted by the evaluator. The person may also be asked to tell the evaluator a story based on the pictures he has drawn.

The Thematic Apperception Test (TAT) was developed by Henry Murray and Christiana D. Morgan in the 1930s at Harvard. It is comprised of cards with pictures that are black and white or in grayscale. These pictures do not have clear meanings and are open to interpretation. Each picture has a theme bearing a relationship to psychoanalytic theory. The person being tested tells a story about each picture, including what leads up to the events in the picture, what is presently happening, and how the story will end. It is believed that unconscious thoughts, feelings, and emotions will come to consciousness and are then able to be interpreted by the analyst. Subjective tests are still in use today.

Psychological testing has become a mainstay in clinical settings, the courts, industry, and research labs. Testing cannot replace a comprehensive interview but is being utilized more to aid in diagnosing and planning an effective treatment plan. If you are being treated and are asked to take a psychological test, educate yourself about the test, and discuss all aspects of it with your clinician. If your child is going to be tested be sure to explain everything to your child to ease his or her fears.

Children and Testing

If your child is experiencing anxiety and it is affecting his or her personal life and school performance you will want to have your child assessed by a mental health practitioner. A comprehensive assessment will be given including in-depth interviews to determine symptoms, family history, present stressors, etc. The clinician might also request permission to administer any number of psychological tests. Your child may start out with an IQ test, and then be asked to take tests like the Beck Youth Inventories created for children ages seven to fourteen. The self-reporting Beck tests contain statements that are answered either true or false and assess symptoms that include symptoms of anxiety and depression, feelings, and emotions. The Revised Children's Manifest Anxiety Scale (RCMAS), developed from the MMPI, is used in schools, clinical settings, and for research purposes to measure symptoms and feelings to be used in diagnosis and creation of treatment plans. Another test is the Social Phobia and Anxiety Inventory (SPAI-C) used to evaluate the child's physical symptoms such as rapid heartbeat, sweaty hands, and shaking in a variety of situations that cause fear and anxiety.

Many tests are self-reporting, but others for younger children are read to the child by the teacher or mental health evaluator. Some tests are given individually, but others can be administered in group situations. A number of tests like the Behavior Rating Inventory of

Executive Function (BRIEF) have a separate questionnaire for parents to fill out about their child.

Testing can be very stressful and anxiety producing for your child. It is important to prepare your child to allay his fears and make him feel as comfortable as possible. Tell your child that he cannot "fail" this test. It is a way to help him. Give your child as much detail as possible about what will happen at the test site and during the test. Try to visit the test site with your child prior to the test. If possible schedule the test at a time that your child functions well. Let your child know he can ask questions about anything, such as results, and will have his questions answered. Some children also feel that something is "wrong" with them because they are being tested. Address this with your child and doctor.

Fact

Psychological testing is done in clinical settings, but much of the testing is done by researchers who are studying a specific subject or disorder on groups of people called subjects or respondents. The results are used to gather data to determine why anxiety disorders develop and to look for more effective forms of treatment.

What Does "Standardization" Mean?

Standardization means that whenever the test is given the content, conditions, scoring, etc., have to be as close to the same for every person. Standardized tests are ordinarily objective tests with questions such as "true" or "false" and contain no essays. To standardize a test, the test has to be given over time to many people, and the results have to be studied by experts. Then revisions are made to improve the test. The test is then given again and the whole process repeats itself until test results prove to be unvarying and average scores or norms have been verified.

Scoring for standardized tests has very specific instructions that must be followed so that any person scoring a test will come up with the same score as anyone else who scores the same test. Scoring is interpreted in comparison to an established "norm" or average for a similar group of people. For example, intelligence tests are scored against the average intelligence of "100." So, if you score above 100, you are considered above average in intelligence, and if you score below 100, you are rated as below average. Norms are created when a test is in the process of being designed. The test is given to a large sample population with similar characteristics. The sample population scores are added up and then divided by the number of people who took the test—that number becomes the average score, or "norm." But it's not as easy as it sounds. Standardized tests are designed, norms are established, and scores are interpreted by using complex statistical methods.

The History of Psychological Testing

In today's world testing is a matter of fact. From your first day of school, all the way thru adulthood, you will be evaluated, rated, and ranked against other people for intelligence, aptitude, personality, etc. With the advent of the Internet it is possible to take thousands of self-administered tests in the attempt to find out about yourself. But testing is not a product of modern mankind, for it has been going on for thousands of years. Testing goes back to the ancient Chinese (2200 B.C.), who tested the abilities of officials.

Written exams covering a variety of subjects such as geography and law have been found in China dating from 202 B.C.–A.D. 200. It was in the 1800s that testing lead to the psychological tests we do today. During that period in time, there arose an interest in how people who were called "mentally retarded or mentally ill" were diagnosed and treated and the differences between the two, which eventually led to the first intelligence tests. By the end of the 1800s tests were designed to evaluate people who were mentally ill or had suffered a brain injury. It was Francis Galton whose interest in "eugenics" led him to develop a series of mental tests with the goal to test human intelligence.

James McKeen Cattell a psychologist with an interest in introducing experimental measurement into psychology as well as developing tests to evaluate intelligence coined the term "mental test." At the turn of the twentieth century, Francis Alfred Binet and Theodore Simon developed the Simon-Binet Intelligence Scale to determine what to do with children who would not benefit from public education. In 1916 Lewis M. Terman from Stanford University revised the Simon-Binet Scale and it became known as the Stanford-Binet Intelligence Test still in use today.

Fact

Eugenics comes from the Greek meaning "well born." It refers to selective breeding in both animals and humans to improve hereditary traits in children. Eugenics has a long history in the United States. For example, in the 1880s laws were passed prohibiting people who were epileptic or considered "feeble-minded" from marrying, and similar state laws existed throughout the 1960s. During World War II the Nazi's used eugenics to attempt to create an Aryan society.

During World War I testing came into its own when the military did psychological testing on large populations of recruits. During World War II intelligence testing as well as aptitude of candidates for pilots was done. The Stanford-Binet Intelligence Test had many critics and in 1939 David Wechsler developed a new IQ test, The Wechsler Adult Intelligence Scale (WAIS)—the most commonly used IQ test today. The MMPI developed in 1930 and revised in 1989 is one of the most widely used objective personality tests today. Projective personality tests such as the Rorschach inkblot test, which emerged from Freudian psychoanalysis, and the TAT (Thematic Apperception Test) both were created in the 1930s and are still in use today. As testing and research progressed numerous scales and inventories were developed, and these continue to be used for specific clinical symptoms and disorders tests such as the Panic Attack Symptoms Questionnaire (PASQ), 1990, and the Agoraphobic Cognitions Scale (ACS), 1992.

Aspects of a Psychological Test

The first psychological tests were created to measure intelligence and aptitude, but as psychological theory changed and testing became acceptable and widespread throughout schools, in health care, industry, and the courts, tests were designed to measure many aspects of human behavior. Designing a psychological test is extremely difficult because the human phenomena being measured, such as personality or aptitude, are not tangible or easily observable and are extremely difficult to measure. The foundations of a good psychological test are reliability and validity. A test is reliable when it can be repeated over and over and get the same results, and scores do not vary. A test is considered valid when it accurately measures what the inventor intended it to. To meet the standards of validity a test must prove to be reliable. But though a test is proven reliable does not necessarily mean it is valid—measuring what it is supposed to.

To make tests reliable and valid, experts distinguished types of reliability and validity the person designing a psychological test must test for, such as test-retest reliability and inter-rater reliability. All tests contain the possibility of error, so a measurement error is added to the true score. Measurement errors might occur for a variety of reasons, which include; the person taking the test was not at their best, maybe anxious, sick, etc. Or the environment was not ideal for test taking, for example, people making noise in the room. Types of validity include face validity and construct validity.

Reliability

To evaluate a test's reliability the test-retest system is used, which means the test was given to the same group of individuals two or more times. Their scores from the first test are compared to the second set of scores to see what changes have occurred. To check for reliability a researcher has to figure out if the differences in scores resulted from the measurement error or from the real scores. Inter-rater reliability examines the scores between people who rate or code tests.

Validity

Researchers question a test's face validity by asking if, on the surface, the test measures what is was designed for. Construct validity is considered the most important type of validity, because it means that the test does measure what it is supposed to. Construct validity is very difficult to achieve and takes a long time.

Generalizability

The word generalizability is often used as an umbrella for reliability and validity in determining if a test is designed well. The term refers to the question of whether a test given to one group of people will show similar results if it is given to another group of people. Or will the results of a test be similar to other tests measuring the same thing. So, will two different intelligence tests get similar results from the same group? And will one test get similar results from two different groups?

Fact

The majority of psychological tests used by clinicians are published by a publisher who specializes in tests. These tests are copyrighted and cannot be copied without permission of the publisher. Your mental health provider has to buy psychological tests from the publishers, which is one of the reasons you have to pay additional fees for the testing.

When Is a Test Invalid?

There are many reasons that will determine whether a test is valid or invalid. Most importantly is test reliability. If the test yields inconsistent scores—when it is repeated many times and scores vary widely—it is considered invalid. Secondly, the person taking the test may slant their answers in a particular way for any number of reasons, which include: inclination for the person taking the test to say "yes" or agree to most of the questions, but the person also may not understand what is being asked; the person taking the test answers questions in such a way that they will look good; the person taking the test says "no" or answers to look bad intentionally for reasons such as getting some kind of compensation.

Cultural bias will invalidate a test if the questions do not have the same meaning across cultures. Face validity, the actual content of the test, may have different meanings to people from other cultures. Bias in the test will occur if the test is measuring a specific quality and the test content is slanted to favor one group over another, such as racial and gender differences. Many tests measure future performance (predictive validity), and experts believe that many tests inaccurately assess performance for minority groups and women. The reasons given for invalidity are also ones that many critics of standardized tests give in their arguments against psychological testing.

Information Revealed in a Clinical Anxiety Test

To diagnose for an anxiety disorder a clinician needs a broad spectrum of information, including your present state, family history, etc. Many tests have been developed to assess the following information:

- Your symptoms will be measured to see if they meet the criteria for an anxiety disorder.
- Are you exhibiting avoidance behavior and, if so, the degree of severity.
- What is the level of your disability in functioning in everyday life?
- Is there a history of anxiety and panic from childhood or in your family?
- Have you experienced significant stressors or traumatic life events?
- Your responses will help the clinician distinguish the kind of anxiety you experience to plan an effective treatment program.
- An evaluation of your coping skills will be done.

- An assessment of the amount of stress you are under will be done to determine if you are at high risk for an anxiety disorder.
- The test will look for other conditions and disorders, for example, depression and substance abuse.

Some health care providers may also administer personality test like the MMPI. Sometimes a test or measurement is given at the beginning of treatment, repeated during treatment to see what progress is being made, and given a third time when treatment is ending. The differences are valuable for the clinician and for the client to see how far he or she has come.

Reasons for Testing

Some mental health practitioners feel that testing can uncover material that is not being made available from their client in the initial stages of treatment. If you are beginning treatment it may be difficult to talk about your problems with a stranger, or you may be ashamed of your feelings, or you may not have enough insight into what is happening with you. The mental health provider may then find it tough to make a diagnosis and set up treatment. Other reasons for testing include:

- Many tests are constructed to tell the evaluator when the person is not giving truthful answers. Objective tests are designed to do this. The evaluator can "red flag" certain responses and uncover the "truth" of the situation later. Subjective tests are used to uncover a person's feelings, attitudes, and experiences, have right or wrong answers, but present material for therapy.
- Proponents of psychological testing, especially objective testing, say it allows the evaluator to make a faster diagnosis based on scientific information rather than doing a series of interviews over weeks or months.

- Some mental health practitioners only do testing for other therapists, the courts, etc. Many are more comfortable with testing and want a quick way to make a diagnosis. Some practitioners may lack good interviewing skills, so giving the client a self-reporting questionnaire is easier for them.

If you decide to enter treatment for your anxiety and are asked to take psychological tests, discuss with your practitioner the reason for the testing, what the test will be assessing and why, and what to expect the test to be like, for example, objective or subjective, time involved, etc. Testing is most likely done by psychologists and sometimes psychiatrists who are specially trained in how to administer tests, to read and write up the results, and then make evaluations, assessments, and diagnoses based on the information.

CHAPTER 14

Medications That Treat Anxiety Disorders

Beginning in the 1950s, medications that eased the symptoms of emotional disorders were developed. Today, medications are often the first type of treatment prescribed. Presently, there are a host of drugs used for the treatment of anxiety disorders, such as tranquilizers and antidepressants. As mentioned earlier, a multidimensional approach to treating anxiety is best, possibly including therapy, lifestyle changes, and other methods as well as medication. This chapter describes the most common drugs in use, along with their side effects.

Psychotropic Medications

We live in an anxious age and use more drugs to alleviate anxiety than other kinds of treatment. Psychotropic drugs are medications used to treat mental illnesses and emotional disorders. These drugs are chemicals that change a person's feelings, emotions, awareness, and thoughts and, in doing so, alter behavior and mental performance. As you read in Chapter 1, medications replaced other means of controlling people such as those who were seriously mentally ill with disorders like schizophrenia, and were controlled by the use of restraints.

Psychotropic drugs did not become prominent until the 1950s, but by the 1960s the chemical revolution was in full swing. The 1980s to the present time has seen an increase in medication for the less serious mental disorders such as anxiety and depression, and presently new drugs come onto the market with increasing speed, or older drugs are approved by the FDA for new uses, for example, Paxil, an antidepressant, has been approved for panic disorder.

What Are the Psychotropic Drugs?

A number of drugs are prescribed today for the treatment of anxiety disorders in the following classifications: benzodiazepines (BZDs) used primarily as anti-anxiety medications and to aid sleep. Tricyclic antidepressants are earlier drugs that help with depressive symptoms and panic disorder. Monoamine oxcidase inhibitors (MAOIs) are also used for depression and anxiety disorders. Serotonin reuptake inhibitors (SSRIs) are used for depression but are effective in treating anxiety disorders like social phobia. Beta-blockers are used to treat hypertension but effective in treating social phobia. Anticonvulsants treat epilepsy but have been prescribed for a number of anxiety disorders. Azaspirones are used to treat anxiety.

Essential

In the 1990s, the numbers of prescriptions written for psychotropic drugs rose exponentially. Studies show, that between 1965–1985, 1.5 billion prescriptions were written for tranquilizers in the United States. In 1997, more than 18 million prescriptions for tranquilizers were filled. Today, more than 60 million prescriptions are written annually for the antidepressants Prozac, Zoloft, and Paxil.

Thinking about Taking Medication?

If you are experiencing the symptoms of anxiety, and are thinking about using medication, the most important thing to do is get an accurate diagnosis. As we have suggested in previous chapters, see your family physician first to rule out physical causes for your symptoms. Then ask to be referred to a psychiatrist who will do a diagnostic evaluation, and prescribe psychotropic medication if necessary. Though you are prescribed medications, there is no guarantee that they will work for you, and your physician may have to change your dosage, or switch you to another drug.

Benzodiazepines

The groups of drugs called benzodiazepines are tranquilizers and sleeping pills and are used to treat anxiety disorders, especially panic attacks, and sleep related problems. Benzodiazepines work by suppressing the central nervous system, leading to the lessening of feelings of anxiety. They are fast acting drugs but are recommended for short-term use due to their addictive qualities. These are often used by people who suffer from severe anxiety for years, which leads to addiction.

 Fact

Commonly known benzodiazepines are: Ativan (lorazepam), Xanax (alprazolam), Klonopin (clonazepam), Valium (diazepam), Librium (chlordiazepoxide), Restoril (temazepam), Halcion (triazolam). Women who are planning to become pregnant, who are pregnant, or want to nurse must see their physician before taking benzodiazepines.

Benzodiazepines are usually taken orally, absorbed in the stomach and small intestine, then metabolized by the liver. They are expelled by the body through urine, excrement, sweating, saliva, and breast milk. Benzodiazepines act on the brain quickly and affect emotions, memory, thinking, awareness, and coordination. These drugs increase the activity of the neurotransmitter, gamma-aminobutyric acid (GABA), whose function is to inhibit or slow down activity, which causes feelings of being calm, and a reduction in stress and anxious feelings.

Side Effects of Benzodiazepines

The down side of benzodiazepines is the risk of becoming dependent with long-term use, and experiencing side effects. Taking these medications for short periods of time, or on occasion when anxiety is severe, will usually not cause the more severe effects. Xanax, one of the most popular of the drugs prescribed, can be highly addictive.

Even a few months of high doses or lower doses taken more than a few months can create physical dependency.

Withdrawal from Benzodiazepines

Withdrawal from benzodiazepines can be as difficult as it is for someone trying to withdraw from heroin. And physical, psychological, and behavioral changes may begin when you try to cut down or skip a dose. The list of withdrawal symptoms numbers over fifty and includes: severe anxiety, agoraphobia, depression, blurred vision, dizziness, irritability, respiratory difficulties, feelings of unreality, extreme lethargy, memory loss, panic attacks, stomach pain/cramps/ nausea, severe headaches, shaking, and heart palpitations.

Essential

If you wish to withdraw from benzodiazepines, contact your doctor for help. You must reduce the dose by taking a little less every day. This will allow your body to adjust to each reduction in dosage and gradually return to normal drug free functioning. Full withdrawal can take weeks, months, and, in some rare cases, years.

Classifications of Benzodiazepines

Benzodiazepines are classified as short, medium, and long acting, referring to how long the drug acts on the body. For example, Halcion, often prescribed for sleeping, acts quickly and does not stay very long in the body—under eight hours. Xanax is a shorter acting drug too, but Valium is a long-acting drug and can stay in the body more than twenty-four hours. The length of drug action is dependent upon a number of factors, your age, weight, and health of your liver.

Long-Term Use

Long-term use of benzodiazepines has shown to increase the possibility of emotional problems, and there is a high risk of developing depression. Cognitive impairment and memory loss have been reported, especially in older populations, and less common but more severe symptoms may include blackouts and hair loss. Stopping benzodiazepines "cold turkey" can cause unbearable pain and distress and may result in "fits or seizures."

Tricyclic Antidepressants

There are three groups of antidepressants, and though each work similarly, they do have differences in their actions and side effects. The tricyclics are older drugs, and though thought to be as effective as the newer SSRIs, they are reported to have more side effects. Used to treat depressive disorders, tricyclics have also been prescribed for panic disorder, social phobia, agoraphobia without panic disorder, and to ease the nightmares of posttraumatic stress disorder.

Tricyclic was first used extensively in the 1950s, and the first drug, Tofranil (imipramine) is still one of the most prescribed tricyclics. Your doctor will start you off with a small dose, to see if any side effects occur and to allow your body to adjust slowly to the drug. Tricyclics work by impeding the deactivation of two neurotransmitters, norepinephrine and serotonin, in the central nervous system. These neurotransmitters are involved in feelings of well-being and activity, and tricyclics allow them to remain active longer in the body.

Tricyclics do not "cure" you of depression or anxiety, or give you a "high," but when they do kick in, usually within a few weeks, you'll find that the severity of your anxiety and depression will lift, and you may feel that you are able to function in areas of your life that you couldn't before beginning the medication. People who do well on a course of treatment with tricyclics report being able to sleep better and experience a decrease in dreaming, feel more energetic, and have an increased ability to concentrate.

Side Effects of Tricyclics

The usual course of treatment on tricyclics is six to eight months. At the beginning of treatment, however, when your body is adjusting to the medication, increases in anxiety, sweating, or night sweats may occur. The main complaint is feeling sedated. Restlessness, problems with falling asleep, or disturbed sleep, and decrease in concentration are common. These symptoms will pass, but many people find them so uncomfortable, they are unable to continue the medication. However, if they do stop abruptly, depression and anxiety may return. Other side effects that cause discomfort and distress include: dry mouth or eyes, having a "funny" taste in your mouth, sensitivity to light, blurry vision, constipation and difficulty urinating, weight gain, and erectile dysfunction.

 Alert

Tricyclics can cause rapid heartbeat, palpitations, or dizziness upon rising. If you have cardiovascular disease, tricyclics can have serious effects on you. They may cause arrhythmias, or worsening of or even causing angina, heart failure, or a heart attack. If you have heart problems, or there is a history of heart problems in your family, before you begin tricyclics, make sure you are checked out by a cardiologist first.

Withdrawal from Tricyclics

Unlike benzodiazepines, tricyclics are not addictive, so you will not develop a dependency, and feel the need to increase your dose to stop symptoms of withdrawal. But problems can ensue if you stop the medication suddenly. If you want to stop taking a tricyclic it is best to do it gradually with the help of your physician. The withdrawal can be uncomfortable, with symptoms that include: feeling anxious and depressed, stomach problems, feeling dizzy, and headaches.

Monoamine Oxidase Inhibitors (MAOIs)

MAOIs work in a similar fashion as tricyclics and the newer SSRIs by their affect on the neurotransmitters serotonin and norepinephrine, but they also act on dopamine, a neurotransmitter in the brain that influences movement. MAOIs block the decrease of these neurotransmitters, called monoamines, whose low levels cause depression. The common names of MAOIs are: Marplan (isocarboxazid), Nardil (phenelzine), and Parnate (tranylcypromine).

The downside to MAOIs is that at the same time that they block the destruction of monamines, levels of another neurotransmitter, tyramine, is increased, which creates an instant rise in blood pressure, which can burst blood vessels in the brain, causing death. Though it is rare, it can happen.

Foods to Avoid on MAOIs

Certain foods have small doses of tryamine. Eating those foods, coupled with the drug, can lead to an overdose and serious side effects. Foods to avoid are: alcoholic beverages, especially wines, sherry, liqueurs, and beer; sausages; pepperoni; salami; bologna; cheeses, especially aged varieties; chicken livers; figs, fruits, such as raisins, bananas, any overripe fruit; meat tenderizer; smoked or pickled meat; poultry and fish; and soy sauce.

 Fact

Because of the potential for death due to an overdose, MAOIs are not a good choice for people with a high risk for suicide, who might intentionally overdose. People with heart problems, epilepsy, asthma, or high blood pressure have to be careful taking MAOIs. And if you get agitated or hyper easily, these drugs may be too stimulating.

Additional Information

Foods that can only be eaten occasionally and in moderation are: avocados, caffeine, chocolate, raspberries, sauerkraut, any commercial soup, sour cream, and yogurt. The diet is so restrictive and difficult to follow that many people find it impossible to stay on MAOIs, though it may be the only medication that has helped their depression. For that reason, and the danger of the drop in blood pressure, most doctors prescribe the newer SSRIs first, and MAOIs only if other antidepressants do not work. Another problematic side effect is the level of sedation; people report they feel like "zombies" on this medication, but many people do adjust and get good results on MAOIs.

Additional Side Effects of MAOIs

In addition to food restrictions and other problems, MAOIs have similar side effects as tricyclics and other antidepressants. The symptoms include: manic states, sedation, dizziness/fainting, sexual problems/low libido, nausea, and weight gain. MAOIs can be very effective in individuals who are depressed and also present with panic attacks.

Children and MAOIs

Children and adolescents are often prescribed antidepressants, but MAOIs are not recommended for children under sixteen, because the drugs are so risky, and studies show they slow growth. Because of the potential for a spike in blood pressure, people older than sixty are not prescribed MAOIs. Remember that in taking any medication, each person has a unique experience, and listed symptoms may not occur. A consult with your doctor will help you decide if MAOIs are best for you.

Selective Serotonin Reuptake Inhibitors (SSRIs)

Selective Serotonin Reuptake Inhibitors (SSRIs) are a group of antidepressants that came on the U.S. market in the 1980s, beginning with Prozac (fluoxetine). This group of drugs is different chemically than the tricyclics and MOAIs, for their only function is to help the brain maintain certain levels of the neurotransmitter serotonin. Researchers believe that low levels of serotonin are involved in the development of depression and some anxiety disorders, such as panic disorder, and that SSRIs will reduce the symptoms of these mental disorders.

SSRIs have shown themselves to be effective for people with depression, panic disorder, social phobia, and obsessive-compulsive disorder. They do not have as many side effects as the older antidepressants, because they do not affect other neurotransmitters, like the MAOIs do. Like all antidepressants, they are not addicting, and there are no withdrawal symptoms, unless they are stopped abruptly, and then the individual may experience flu-like symptoms, such as, headaches and body pain. Commonly known SSRIs are:

- *Fluoxetine*: Prozec, Fontex, Seromex, Seronil, Sarafem
- *Paroxetine*: Paxil, Seroxat, Optipar, Aropax, Paroxat
- *Sertraline*: Zoloft
- *Citalopram*: Celexa, Cipramil, Emocal, Sepram
- *Fluvoxamine maleate*: Luvox, Faverin

Fact

David Healy, a psychiatrist and former secretary of the British Association for Psychopharmacology, wrote *Let Them Eat Prozac* (2004). Healy, who prescribed Prozac to his patients, began to see troubling symptoms in many of his patients and believes that the pharmaceutical industry hid the clinical trial data because of the profit motive. He states that all trial data should be made public knowledge.

Children and SSRIs

SSRIs have been prescribed for children and adolescents, but in 2004, the Federal Drug Administration (FDA) issued a public health warning that stated that antidepressants, targeting SSRIs, in children and adults may bring on suicidal thoughts and attempts if the individual is being treated for depression. The FDA information does not mention if individuals using SSRIs for anxiety are more likely to have a higher risk for suicide. Pharmaceutical companies have been asked to add warnings to their labels.

Additional Information

One of the problems with SSRIs, as opposed to tricyclics, MAOIs, and benzodiazepines, is that SSRIs can take a long time, from four to six weeks, for the person to notice a change in how they feel. Also, as you begin to take an SSRI, you may feel a temporary increase in anxiety. Other side effects include the following, but usually subside as your body adjusts: dry mouth, tremors, diarrhea, loss of appetite, nausea, headaches, insomnia, feeling drowsy, fatigue, confusion, and sexual difficulties. But like older antidepressants, as your body adjusts to the drug, symptoms usually abate.

Beta-Blockers

Beta-Blockers are beta-adrenergic blocking agents, commonly used in the treatment of high blood pressure (hypertension). They are also used to prevent a second heart attack, relieve chest pain (angina), stop migraines, and tremors. Beta-blockers work by "blocking" the effects of stress hormones, such as adrenaline, and easing the workload of the heart.

When stress hormones are activated, beta-receptors cause the heart rate to slow and heart muscle contractions to decrease. Beta-receptors are structures that exist on nerve cell membranes of the sympathetic nervous system and affect its activities, such as heart rate. Beta-blockers bind with the beta-receptors and prevent stress hormones from entering the receptors and triggering the stress reaction. It is because of this effect on stress hormones that the "fight or flight" reaction does not kick in, so the symptoms of anxiety, such as racing heart and sweating, do not manifest themselves. Common beta-blockers include:

- Inderal-LA (propranolol)
- Lopressor (metoprolol)
- Betapace (sotalol)
- Normodyne (labetalol)
- Trandate (labetalol)
- Sectral (acebutolol)

Beta-blockers are often prescribed for people who have social phobia, because it reduces the more noticeable signs of anxiety, such as shaking, trembling, and blushing. Individuals who experience performance anxiety, such as public speakers and performers, also use these. Beta-blockers have been called "the underground drug" for musicians, because it helps to stop the symptoms of performance anxiety, which include thought blocking and loss of concentration. Beta-blockers do not in any way influence the emotional component of anxiety—they only have a physiological effect and can usually stop the "fight or flight" reaction from starting. Though, if anxiety is high enough, beta-blockers may not be able to reduce the symptoms enough to feel relief. Beta-blockers are not addicting and begin to work within a few hours after swallowing and come in either tablet or liquid form.

Side Effects of Beta-Blockers

Beta-blockers have side effects especially within the first few weeks of treatment. You may not experience any symptoms but if you do they may include: fatigue, cold extremities, upset stomach, sleep disturbances/nightmares, dizziness/feeling lightheaded and faint, wheezing/chest feels tight, and skin rashes.

Fact

Since beta-blockers act quickly, they can be taken on an as needed basis for anxiety. It is recommended that 20 to 40 milligrams of a beta-blocker, such as propranolol (Inderal), is taken one hour before the stressful situation. If your anxiety is very high, and the beta-blocker will not give you enough relief, then you can usually safely combine it with a benzodiazepine, such as alprazolam (Xanax). Remember, you must check with your doctor before combining medications.

If taken occasionally, beta-blockers usually have no side effects. Even if taken daily, they are not associated with weight gain or sexual problems, but males taking higher doses have reported difficulties in achieving erection. If you are taking beta-blockers on a daily basis for more than a month, and you want to stop, it is best to stop gradually. Though you will not experience withdrawal symptoms, you may have a very high spike in blood pressure. Another caution is the use of alcohol, which can only exacerbate the effects of sedation, and also lower blood pressure.

Azaspirones

Azaspirones are a group of anti-anxiety drugs, used to a variety of anxiety disorders. The most common of the azaspirones is BuSpar, shown to be an effective treatment of mild to moderate symptoms of anxiety. Azaspirones normally take two to four weeks before their effectiveness kicks in and are not considered to be addictive with potential for abuse. BuSpar influences the neurotransmitters dopamine, norepinephrine, and serotonin and acts on calming emotions. Side effects are usually mild and go away within a few weeks but may be more severe and include:

- Drowsiness
- Fatigue
- Nausea
- Feeling hyper
- Depression
- Insomnia
- Feeling lightheaded

Azaspirones are used to reduce the symptoms of obsessive-compulsive disorder, and general anxiety disorder. Rare symptoms include: chest pains, muscle weakness, rashes, uncontrolled movements, increase in blood pressure, and tremors. Overdose is possible and those symptoms are: dizziness, fainting, nausea or vomiting, and unconsciousness. If you experience any severe symptoms, see your doctor immediately, or go to the nearest emergency room.

Anticonvulsants

Anticonvulsants are a group of drugs that are ordinarily used to treat diseases, like epilepsy, because they stop seizures and fits. Their use has been expanded to the treatment of mood disorders, such as bipolar disorder. And recent research has indicated their usefulness in the treatment of anxiety disorders, such as generalized anxiety disorder, social phobia, posttraumatic stress disorder, and panic disorder. Anticonvulsants work by reducing abnormal activity of certain nerves in the brain and the way they do so differs with each medication.

Common anticonvulsants include:

- Divalproex sodium (Depakote)
- Felbamate (Felbatol)
- Gabapentin (Neurontin)
- Lamotrigine (Lamictal)
- Topiramate (Topamax)
- Tiagabine (Gabitril)
- Carbamazepine (Tegretol)

Alert

If you are taking anticonvulsants for at least a few months and want to stop, do not quit cold turkey. Abruptly stopping can cause seizures, especially if you have a seizure disorder or bipolar disorder. All anticonvulsants need to be withdrawn gradually. Slowly withdrawing from these drugs may cause dizziness, confusion, and sensitivity to light and sound. Always discuss stopping a medication with your physician.

The side effects of anticonvulsants can be difficult to cope with, but at low doses, there is a good chance that the effects will be mild. Reactions include lethargy and becoming very sensitive to sunlight. Mood swings are common, and they also slow down metabolism, so weight gain can be an issue. Memory and cognitive processes can be affected negatively, especially short-term memory loss. This group of drugs seems to impact dreams and has been used to reduce the nightmares associated with posttraumatic stress disorder. Skin rashes are common, as are acne and fungal infections. Anticonvulsants can cause gums to bleed and maybe weaken the enamel on teeth, and cause thinning hair. A rare side effect is the development of aplastic anemia, a potentially deadly disease.

Guidelines for Taking Medication

Medications can be effective in treating your anxiety disorder, but to get the most out of them, and to keep yourself safe, you want to follow a few rules:

- Proper diagnosis is necessary to create a successful treatment plan.
- Tell your physician about any physical or mental conditions, other medications, herbs, and supplements, or other relevant information about yourself.
- Educate yourself about your condition and what drugs and other treatments have shown to be effective.
- Know what you can expect from your medication as far as relieving your condition, and its side effects.
- Report all changes and side effects immediately to your doctor.
- Do not deviate from the recommended dosage.
- If you want to stop, do not do so without the supervision of your physician.
- Children and elderly people require special attention with regard to the effects of medication.
- Drug therapy works best when combined with counseling or psychotherapy.

Medication is only one part of a successful treatment plan. There is no "miracle" drug that will cure anxiety disorders. Many people with anxiety disorders do not choose to take medication because of the side effects and use other means to overcome their conditions. But there is no shame in taking medications, and you are not "weak" if you choose to do so. Discuss your feelings, fears, etc., about medications openly with your physician and with his or her help come up with the best solution for treating your anxiety.

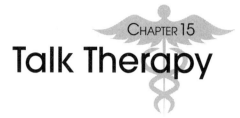

CHAPTER 15

Talk Therapy

Talk therapy is an effective treatment for anxiety disorders and other emotional conditions. Going into therapy for the first time may feel uncomfortable or even frightening. But once you learn what talk therapy is, who does it, and what to expect from a session, it will lose its mystery. This chapter describes some of the many therapies available, providing information you need to choose the right therapy path for you.

What Is Talk Therapy?

Talk therapy has been around as long as people have had language. When things bother us we often feel better when we "talk things out" with someone, whether it be a family member, friend, religious person, or a therapist. Working with a therapist can help you with emotional problems, and to sort out difficulties you are having in life. You can become more aware of your feelings and how you are behaving. It's helpful to get someone else's perspective on what is bothering you, and have someone in your corner who listens and supports you. And it just feels good to have someone listen intently to how you feel. Talk therapy is also called counseling, therapy, psychotherapy, and psychoanalysis.

Psychotherapy can be short-term, lasting weeks or months. Long-term therapy may continue for many years. Most therapists meet with clients once a week or twice a month. But Freudian psychoanalysis usually requires two or even three meetings per week. There are different methods of therapy that include:

- Individual psychotherapy
- Couples/Marital therapy
- Group psychotherapy
- Family therapy
- Child/Play therapy

Psychotherapy may be the only treatment you receive, or it may be combined with other treatment, like medication, for example. It all depends on your level of distress and diagnosis, for example, if you have been diagnosed with an emotional disorder, and what treatment plan you have discussed with your physician and mental health clinician, and how you feel about entering into a type of treatment.

Fact

In the late nineteenth century Freud, with his "talking cure," set in motion what would become modern day psychotherapy. Talk therapy is essentially a dialogue between a person who is having life problems, with a licensed mental health clinician, who has either a master's degree, a Ph.D., or an M.D., and is specially trained in one or more psychotherapies.

Who Does Talk Therapy?

If you are thinking about entering psychotherapy it is important to be able to distinguish between the different credentials that mental health clinicians carry. The type of degree will not tell you the type of therapy the clinician practices, but it will educate you about the person's academic training. Information about experience and what theory base they practice from will require you to do a phone interview or go in for an initial session. The different clinicians are: psychologists, who have studied psychology, and have either a master's degree, which is two years of graduate work, or a doctorate, which is at least four years of graduate work. Degrees include: Ph.D. (Doctor of Philosophy); Psy.D. (Doctor of Psychology); and Ed.D. (Doctor of Education).

Clinicians with doctorates are qualified to be licensed. Psychologists may also have a master's degree (M.S. or M.A.) that requires two years of graduate school and are also eligible for licensing.

Social Workers have studied clinical social work, or social work policy. They may have a doctorate or master's in social work that required four years or two years, respectively, of graduate school. Degrees include: D.S.W. (Doctor of Social Work); M.S.W. (Master's of Social Work); A.C.S.W. (Academy of Certified Social Workers); D.C.S.W. (Diploma of Clinical Social Work), a five year post graduate credential; L.S.W. (Licensed Social Worker); L.C.S.W. (Licensed Clinical Social Worker). Most states require clinicians to be licensed. Marriage and family therapists/professional counselors have studied family systems, psychology, and counseling. Degrees include: M.A. (Master of Arts); M.S. (Master of Science); M.Ed. (Master of Education). Psychiatrists are medical doctors (M.D.) with a specialty in psychiatry. After college they go to medical school. Some psychiatrists only do evaluations for mental illnesses and conditions and prescribe medication, but many also do some type of psychotherapy.

Essential

Many mental health providers call themselves psychotherapists, which is a reference to the kind of work they do, "psychotherapy." Any mental health provider can be a psychotherapist, including psychologists, social workers, or counselors. Look for someone with at least a master's degree in psychology/human behavior, who is licensed, and has experience treating your type of problem.

Depending on state law, not all clinicians have to be licensed to practice, so you want to find a therapist who is licensed. Licensing tells you that the therapist has the necessary education and training, and must continue to educate and train to maintain a current license. Licensed therapists have a state board that they must answer to and must practice within a code of ethics. Also, therapy by a licensed mental health provider may be covered by insurance.

How to Find and Choose a Therapist

Therapy is a collaborative process. And the relationship you develop with your therapist will be vital to your healing and overcoming anxiety. This is the person who you will be telling intimate and maybe painful things to, so you want to feel good about your therapist, that you can trust him or her, and also that you like their approach to your problems. Finding a therapist may require legwork on your part and you may have to try out a number of therapists before you find the one for you. The following are suggestions for finding a therapist:

- Through friends and relatives who have had a good experience in therapy —this is one of the best ways to find a therapist.
- Through your family physician.
- Through your insurance company.
- Through your local mental health association or hospital.
- Through professional associations for mental health providers.
- Through Anxiety Disorders Association of America and other organizations like it.

Once you have gathered a handful of names of therapists, your next step is to call each therapist, describe your symptoms, and tell them what your goals are. Ask them if they have treated the problems you describe and for how long. Also, ask if they are licensed—if your state does not require a license to practice, ask what training they have and what professional associations they belong to. Inquire about how they might go about treating your problem. Finally, don't forget the practical aspects—ask about fees, insurance reimbursement, and office procedures.

If at any time you are not happy with your progress or your therapist, or anything else about the therapeutic process, discuss how you feel with your therapist. A good therapist wants to know how you feel about the therapy, progress you feel you are making, etc., and will not be offended—it is all part of the therapeutic process. If you are not happy with your therapist, and have given it a chance, it may be best to look for another therapist. Remember, too, that therapists work from a code of ethics, and if at any time during therapy you feel uncomfortable with the relationship between you and your therapist, for example, if your therapist makes sexual advances, or does anything else that is unprofessional, then leave immediately and report the occurrence to the state licensing board.

What to Expect from a Therapy Session

Each therapy session has a unique quality to it, as different as the people who are sitting in the room. And each therapist has a different approach and style to the work. The therapist's first goal is to not only find out why you have come into therapy but to build a rapport and trust, so you will feel safe to express yourself without feeling judged or censored. And no matter what the contrast is between therapists and their theories, there are fundamental guidelines that form the structure of a therapy session. Consider the following:

- Prior to your first session, you will decide on the appointment date, time, and fee by telephone.
- After the initial greeting, the therapist will probably write down your contact, and possibly insurance, information. You may be asked to sign relevant forms, such as billing forms, if the therapist does not have an office staff.
- The therapist will ask you why you are seeking therapy. While you are talking the therapist will most likely be writing down what you say at his initial session. (Therapists must keep notes on each session, and all notes and information on you must be kept in a locked file for confidentiality purposes.)
- During the initial session, the therapist will ask questions about family history and your personal history, past experiences, medical history, etc. This probing for information is important, so the therapist can begin to get to know you

better, and have a clearer understanding about why you came in. Your therapist will explain that everything you say in therapy is completely confidential.

- The therapist should mention that you might feel upset talking about personal feelings, events, and circumstances at first, and that this is a normal reaction to beginning therapy. You may not want to continue the discussion or need to withhold information at first, and doing so is okay. It takes time to build trust.

- Depending on why you are in therapy, and what type of therapy you are in, after a few sessions, the therapist may work with you on setting up short-term and long-term therapy goals, and help you to set up a plan for achieving them. Psychotherapy usually involves weekly or at least twice a month meetings.

- For the most part, the client will begin each session with what is important for them at that moment in time. Most therapists do not "lead" the session but rather "guide" the work, because psychotherapy is an empowering process, which helps individuals discover their capacity and capability to have a satisfying and productive life.

No matter what theory base the therapist works in, all good therapy is based on the foundation of building a solid working relationship between client and therapist, so your therapist must have characteristics such as genuineness, warmth and caring, empathy, and open-mindedness.

Deciding to enter into therapy is an important decision that requires effort, time, and money on your part. It is important that you are satisfied with your therapist, feel a rapport, and are comfortable talking about what is troubling you as well as what might come up in each session between you and your therapist.

Does Talk Therapy Work?

The effectiveness of psychotherapy and counseling has been studied extensively over many decades, and research indicates that therapy works. But since psychotherapy is an inexact process it has been difficult to test and prove the results. Early studies testing the efficacy of short-term and long-term therapy on depression and anxiety disorders, in the 1970s and 1980s, found that, within a short period of time from the start of psychotherapy, symptoms lessened. And long-term affects showed less emotional distress and better functioning in every aspect of life.

 ## Fact

By using single photon emission computed tomography (SPECT) imaging experts have demonstrated that psychological therapy can alter responses in the brain. One study showed that panic attacks can be triggered by "lactate infusion" in people with panic disorder. When these same people had a course of cognitive therapy, the lactate-influenced panic attacks were reversed.

Many studies coupled the results with a combination of medication and therapy, but when drugs were discontinued because of side effects, and therapy continued, the results were as good for the nonmedicated individuals. A number of studies show that in looking at overall effectiveness of people in therapy, no one therapeutic theory stands out, but the abilities of the therapist made a positive difference. Another significant finding was that the commitment of the client in working with the therapist in the therapist's orientation has a positive affect on outcome. Advances in science and technology are allowing researchers to come close to scientifically proving that psychotherapy is an effective treatment that definitely affects the neural patterning of the brain with positive results.

Other studies have examined the impact of psychodynamic psychotherapy on levels of serotonin. One researcher showed that after one year of psychotherapy, SPECT imaging revealed that those subjects had normal amounts of serotonin, while the subjects with reduced levels of serotonin had no psychotherapy. Thoughts are that psychotherapy may normalize levels of serotonin, but more studies are continuing. What is agreed on by experts is that psychotherapy is an effective treatment for emotional problems, whether as a stand alone treatment or in combination with other treatment, such as medication. The remainder of the chapter will list and discuss some of these therapies.

Behavior Therapy

Behavior therapy is a melding of the application of the principles of learning theory to the analysis and treatment of behavior. It involves more than principles of learning and uses the empirical findings of social and experimental psychology. The emphasis is upon the client's present behavior that is causing distress and disruption in the client's life. The therapist's job is to observe the client's behavior, discuss the maladaptive patterns of behavior with the client, and help the client to go about changing the behavior.

The client's past history, feelings, emotional states, and unresolved experiences are not the focus of the work. If working with a client who has specific phobias, graded exposure, or a systematic desensitization program is often created to help the patient enter previously feared situations. The therapist will most likely teach an anxious client relaxation techniques and increase coping skills. There are various behavior therapies.

Dialectical Behavior Therapy (DBT)

Dr. Marsha Linehan developed DBT for patients struggling with chronic suicidal behaviors. It's based on the idea that psychosocial treatment of those with borderline personality disorder (a disorder with symptoms of high anxiety) was as important in controlling the condition as traditional psychotherapy and medication were. Along with this belief came a pattern of treatment goals. Foremost among these was reducing self-injuring/suicidal behavior; following that came decreasing behaviors that interfered with the therapy or treatment process; and finally, downgrading behaviors that lessened the client's quality of life.

Rational-Emotive Therapy

Founded by Albert Ellis, rational-emotive therapy is highly action-oriented and deals with the client's cognitive and ethical state. The therapy emphasizes the client's ability to think on his own, and in his ability to change. The rational-emotive therapist believes that people are born with the ability of rational thinking but that we may fall victim to irrational thinking. The therapist will use directed therapy. The therapist believes that a neurosis is a result of irrational behavior and irrational thinking. The rational-emotive therapist believes the client's problems are rooted in childhood and in his beliefs that were formed early on. Therapy will include method solving and dealing with emotional or behavior problems. The therapist will help the client eliminate any self-defeating outlooks they may have and to view life in a rational way.

Cognitive Behavioral Therapy (CBT)

Cognitive behavioral therapies are a melding of the cognitive therapies that were formulated from cognitive therapy, whose focus is helping people change their thought patterns, and the classical behavioral therapies, such as operant conditioning, where change in behavior is the primary goal. Both therapies emphasize that change can take place without having deep insight into one's behavior. In CBT, it is thinking patterns that cause symptoms. Changing how you think about yourself, your attitudes and beliefs, and the situation you are in will relieve troubling symptoms. Learning how to face life in a confident and calm manner will help to change your behavior. CBT has shown to be effective in treating panic disorders, phobias, chronic anxiety, and worry. It is short-term therapy and cost effective and is the preferred therapy today for treating anxiety and depression, and many other emotional conditions and life problems.

Neuro-Linguistic Programming (NLP)

In the late 1970s, Richard Bandler, a mathematician, and John Grinder, a linguist, collaborated on bringing a new methodology to the discipline of studying and working with human behavior. Based on the advances made in information technology, particularly computer programming, and the science of language, Bandler and Grinder founded NLP techniques that enable you to use your own mind to make changes in your thoughts, attitudes, beliefs, and ultimately emotions and behaviors. These changes, they propose, will stop self-defeating behaviors and enable you to fulfill your life potential.

Fact

Neurosis is an unconscious maladaptive mental condition that causes anxiety, conflicts in life, obsessions, compulsions, and phobias. Freud believed that neurosis was caused by unconscious defense mechanisms used to ward off anxiety due to unconscious conflicts. Neurosis is a term no longer used in the DSM-IV to define mental disorders.

Bandler and Grinder investigated how people experience the world through the five senses: visual (mental images), auditory (sound), kinesthetic (touch and emotions), gustatory (taste), and olfactory (smell). They examined how these experiences become the memories and images we carry around in our heads, and how these mental pictures affect our emotions and behavior. They studied individuals who were successful, unafraid, etc., and analyzed through complex methods how these people interpreted experiences, life events, other people, etc., to account for their positive, capable behavior, compared to others who had negative reactions. Bandler and Grinder then devised techniques that often only take a few minutes, which allow anyone to change negative mental pictures, feelings, and behavior into positive thoughts, emotions, and behavior.

NLP is presently used by people who want to reach high levels of performance; in psychotherapy to treat anxiety, phobias and depression; as a self-help method; and in business and industry to increase productivity and attain success.

Psychotherapy

There are numerous therapies that are called psychotherapy, or are psychodynamically oriented, having evolved out of Freud's psychoanalysis. Basically psychotherapy is helping the client work through thoughts, feelings, emotions, and behaviors that are causing distress and problems in the client's life. All of these therapies focus on the unconscious, and that early childhood experiences play a critical role in the development of personality and behavior. Emphasis is placed on uncovering painful experiences and unresolved feelings and that doing so will increase symptoms and help to change self-defeating behaviors. A main goal of psychodynamic therapy is for the person to fully understand him or herself. The process of psychotherapy includes becoming aware of thoughts, feelings, emotions, accepting and handling emotions and feelings, emotionally releasing fear and guilt, having insight into "self," and experiencing emotional growth.

L. Essential

Many of the psychodynamic psychotherapies are long-term and treatment can last for years, but some have developed into short-term, more solution focused work, but without discarding the emphasis on insight-oriented theories. Part of this change is due to the advent of managed care, whose emphasis is on brief therapy for relief of symptoms, with only a limited number of sessions authorized per year.

Essential to every type of therapy is the relationship with the therapist. The therapist's office is the place where you will reveal yourself emotionally and that can be uncomfortable and painful at times—though it is part of the process of emotional growth. Because of this, it is imperative that you trust your therapist to guide you through this sometimes difficult but also liberating process.

Psychoanalytic Psychotherapy

Psychoanalytic psychotherapy evolved from Freudian psychoanalysis, and its theory is based on the belief that most of our thoughts, behaviors, and attitudes are controlled by unconscious drives, and are not in our conscious control. The therapist sits out of view of the person, who lies on a couch and talks about anything that comes to mind. The therapist will interact with the client by asking questions, making interpretations, and confronting distorted thinking. The patient's unconscious patterns of thought are "transferred" on to the therapist who interprets this process, thus making the unconscious, conscious. The goal is to help the patient make deep psychic changes. There is an emphasis on the individual's quest for individuation, and finding a sense of identity. Psychoanalytic psychotherapy is thought to be only long-term, but many therapists do short-term work too.

Short-term dynamic therapy (STDT) is based on the same principles as psychoanalytic psychotherapy but differs in the therapist's method of practice and goals. STDT helps the person become aware of how past experiences and present day experiences influence the problems the person has presented in therapy. The therapist will interpret the person's defenses, resistance to therapy, and transference that is causing the person's distressing symptoms. The STDT therapist takes on a more active role than the psychoanalytical psychotherapy therapist. Therapy is usually completed in ten to twenty sessions but may take longer if the patient's problems are severe.

Jungian Analytical Psychotherapy
and Ego Psychology/Ego State Psychotherapy

Given that Jung was a contemporary of Freud, a major role in analytical psychotherapy is the analyst's interpretation of the client's dreams and fantasies used to uncover and recognize what the client has repressed in his or her unconscious, and once the client is aware, symptoms will decrease. Jung's theory also connected the ancient past with the client's present, as he believed that archetypes, which are universal symbols, forms, and patterns that are unconscious and biological, and the collective unconscious, the part of the unconscious that is shared with all humans, were important to the analysis.

Fact

Twenty-four hour therapy is a radical method of confronting clients with "reality" to help them develop self-sufficiency and control over their lives. During the twenty-four hours, the therapist directs a team of trained people to have complete control over the client's physical, social, financial, and sexual life. Therapy can last for weeks to one year and usually takes place in the client's home. This method has led to legal and ethical implications.

Ego psychology's main feature is working on the person's emotional development, and strengthening the ego in the individual. The ego is believed to be a positive force in the development of personality. A weak ego will create an "identity crises." Identity crises are not viewed as negative developments but are seen by the therapist as an opportunity for the client to make positive growth and change. The therapist employs discussion, instruction, teaching, and experiential exercises in the course of therapy.

Client-Centered Therapy and Existential Psychotherapy

Developed by Carl Rogers in the 1940s, client-centered therapy is a nondirective approach. Directive approaches include asking questions, interpreting client's statements/dreams, giving homework, evaluating behavior, etc. Client-centered therapists give total control of the therapy to the client, believing that people are able to find the answers to their problems, and that the therapist is present to understand and accept the client. The basic premise of client-centered therapy is that humans tend toward self-actualization and healthy psychological growth. The therapist helps the client to self-actualize through his or her genuine caring and nonjudgmental understanding of the client.

Existential psychotherapy developed out of the philosophical foundations of existential philosophers such as Sartre and Kierkegaard and was adapted into therapy by humanistic theorists. Modern existentialist therapists are Spinelli and Yalom. The basic theory is that the therapist helps the client to face and accept the following: the anxiety that arises from the reality of being alive, which includes having to face death. Therapists help clients explore their assumptions about life, and learn what is meaningful to them by becoming aware of their emotions and beliefs.

Gestalt Psychotherapy

Gestalt psychotherapy was founded by Friedrick (Fritz) Perls, a humanist therapist. Gestalt therapy believes that emotional disorders are caused by the individual's unconscious needs, wishes, emotions, and obsessions. The Gestalt therapeutic relationship is experiential, in the here and now, and involves various forms of expressive techniques, such as pantomime, role playing, and painting. Through this therapy the person becomes aware of his unconscious, but with healthier, more suitable emotions. Gestalt therapists' focus is on what is happening in the session between client and therapist, rather than content, which opens the door for discussion and experimentation. The goal of therapy is for the client to accept and value himself.

Solution-Focused Brief Therapy (SFBT)

Solution-focused brief therapy is an action-oriented therapy where treatment is often begun and terminated in three to six sessions. Unlike long-term psychotherapy where time is spent on examining past life events and problems, SFBT zeros in on the present and future to help the client with the following:

- What is working in your life?
- What is not working in your life?

- What changes do you want to make?
- What steps have to be taken to make the changes?

SFBT therapy helps the client recognize behaviors that are standing in the way of the life he wants. The therapist also guides the client in setting up short- and long-term goals and aids the client in devising a plan to meet those goals. The SFBT therapist works from a philosophy that the client is the expert about his own life and makes the decisions on the changes to be made. SFBT is used to treat individuals with anxiety, depression, and other mental conditions and disorders.

Eclectic Therapy

Eclectic therapy refers to therapists who use various theoretical orientations and choose a mix of techniques from more than one therapy approach. What results is a mix tailored to the individual. Eclectics use techniques from all schools of therapy, such as what might be reinforcing unhealthy behaviors (behaviorism), unhealthy thoughts (cognitive), and how these all relate to each other in the individual who has come for therapy (humanistic). In eclecticism, there is no one right way of approaching any given problem. The therapist proceeds with the work by being cognizant of the patient's unique view of himself and how he sees his problem, and his world.

Child Play Therapy

When children suffer from emotional problems, therapeutic play is used because children may not be able to cognitively and verbally communicate their feelings and experiences, and play is the way children naturally learn and express themselves. Therapeutic play is adapted to meet the child's developmental needs. Through play therapy children can also learn how to become aware of their behavior and its effect on others, change negative behaviors into positive ones, find solutions to problems, and improve self-confidence and social skills. Play therapy is used to treat behavioral and learning problems, anxiety and depression, stress disorders, ADHD, and other mental and social problems.

Group Therapy

Group therapy is widely practiced today, but for a long time it was regarded as less effective than individual therapy. However, that view appears to be changing. Current research shows the effectiveness of groups that are based around anxiety disorder, depression, relationship problems, and personality disorders. For example, cognitive-behavioral therapy (CBT) is now being utilized by group psychotherapists to unite members with anxiety and mood disorders.

There are many kinds of groups and these differences depend on their goals and the structure and theory base of the therapist. In group therapy, sessions consist of a number of people, usually between six and twelve, and a therapist. Patients learn how to relate to others, and modify their own behavior, see how other members handle life situations and feel supported. Some groups meet around a single issue, such as panic disorder or drug and alcohol abuse. Other groups are general therapy groups, and often members are also working in individual therapy. Groups can be run using almost any psychological theory.

The therapist may refer a client to a group in existence or one that is just forming. The therapist will assess all potential group participants to see if a group is the proper setting for treatment. Groups will not usually work for people in acute crisis, those with a history of poor attendance, people who have difficulties with self-disclosure, and individuals who are disruptive.

Family and Marriage/Couple Therapy

Family therapists view each family as a complex system with a unique way of functioning. Each family has its own way of communicating, roles and rules for each member, and patterns of behavior. Each of us is powerfully affected by our family system. Changes in one member's behavior or emotional problems impact the entire family unit.

Family therapists help families with the following:

- Becoming aware of both the positive and negative patterns of family behavior
- Focus on changes in the entire family not just one member

- Help families set long and short-term goals and create strategies for achieving goals
- Teach members positive ways to communicate with each other
- How to manage and solve conflicts

Family therapy is action-oriented and solution focused. It can be brief therapy or, if problems are severe, can be long term. Besides nuclear family members, extended family members, other individuals important to a particular situation, and even pets may be brought into sessions.

Essential

EMDR (eye movement desensitization and reprocessing), pioneered by Francine Shapiro, is a treatment for posttraumatic stress disorder. In an EMDR session clients are asked to think about the traumatic events repeatedly while following the therapist's index and middle fingers as they quickly move from left to right in front of the client, which will lessen the anxiety.

Marriage and couple therapy is similar to family therapy, but the focus is on the parents or partners. It too is action-oriented and focused on setting long- and short-term goals and developing a plan to achieve them. Couples are often given assignments to complete at home, for example taking time alone to practice new ways to communicate. In both family and marriage/couple therapy members may also be in individual therapy at the same time.

How to Find and Choose a Support Group

Self-help groups offer an important resource for people with anxiety and related problems. Even if you are in therapy you may want to join a support group too. The members of these groups are facing the same issues that you are. Support group members can empathize with your struggle, your problems, and applaud your successes. Being in a support group will also help you feel less isolated.

There are many regional and local self-help groups that deal with anxiety-related problems. It's been estimated that more than 12 million people participate in more than 500,000 self-help groups across the nation. With so large a representation, there's the likelihood that you will find one in your area. The first place to look for a support group is the phone book. If either the white pages or the yellow pages have a listing for "Community Services," look in the table of contents for the heading, "Mental Health." Or check out the "blue" pages under mental health. If you strike out, call your local hospital. Some support groups originate with a therapist in private practice or a mental health clinic. Others will be national, regional, and local self-help groups and may not have a professional facilitator leading the group.

After you have the names of several groups, it's time to choose the one that's right for you. The best way to do that is to attend at least three sessions of each group to see and hear if it's the one for you. Because there's so much at stake, be prepared not only to listen but perhaps ask questions of the moderator after the meeting is over.

If you're unable to find a local self-help group, maybe you should think of forming one yourself. You can't be the only individual in your area, and once it's advertised in the local paper, you'll find others who'll want to join too. You can get help from the nonprofit Anxiety Disorders Association of America. They can assist you in starting up a local support group, or check with your community hospital.

CHAPTER 16

Alternative Treatments and Therapies for Anxiety

Alternative treatments for diseases and emotional distress go back to the beginning of mankind, and the use of herbs, bodywork, energy therapies, etc., as methods of healing are still popular today. Many physicians have incorporated the use of these complimentary treatments in their medical practices. This chapter takes a closer look at the more common alternative treatments and how they help ease anxiety. Note: The information in this chapter is not intended as a substitute for the expertise and advice of your primary health care provider. Always discuss any decisions about treatment or care with your health care provider.

What Does "Alternative" Mean?

Complementary and alternative medicine (CAM) utilizes a wide array of therapies outside of conventional medicine. While there have been scientific studies done for some remedies, in large part questions remain about the majority of the therapies designed to treat diseases or medical conditions. Alternative treatments include the use of herbs, massage, medical philosophy substances, and techniques from other cultures, such as Hindu and Chinese medicine, massage, yoga, and meditation.

Complementary medicine is used together with conventional medicine. Alternative medicine is used instead of conventional medicine. Integrative medicine joins both conventional medicine and CAM therapies, which have scientific evidence of usefulness and safety. An example of complementary medicine is using aromatherapy to help lessen a patient's distress after surgery. An example of alternative therapy is using a special diet to treat cancer instead of undergoing surgery, radiation, or chemotherapy. According to the National Institute of Health there are five "domains" of complementary and alternative medicine.

Alternative Medical Systems and Practitioners

Alternative medical systems are based upon theory and practice. Many of these systems were begun thousands of years before the onset of medical practice. Examples of alternative medicine that developed in Western cultures include homeopathic and naturopathic medicine, which are holistic healing philosophies and use certain substances to treat a variety of ills. Traditional Chinese medicine and Ayurveda were developed in non-Western cultures.

But who are the alternative practitioners? While a number of conventional physicians have been investigating the positive properties of alternative medicine, and recommending them to their patients, it's still a slow go because Western medicine is just beginning to seriously try to incorporate and benefit from the healing wisdom of ancient therapeutics. In the main, the practitioners of the various remedies in alternative medicine are not M.D.s; however, they are usually members of industry associations, which lay down specific guidelines and requirements that their members consent to follow. A consumer seeking an alternative treatment for a problem would be wise to use practitioners who are so allied.

 Fact

The National Institute of Health reports that mind-body interventions constitute a major portion of the overall use of CAM by the public. In 2002, five relaxation techniques and imagery, biofeedback, and hypnosis, taken together, were used by more than 30 percent of the adult U.S. population. Prayer was used by more than 50 percent of the population.

Biologically Based Remedies

Biologically based remedies use materials found in nature, such as herbs and food. For example, it is said that the Five Flower Remedy from Bach Flower Essences gives quick relief from acute anxiety, kava kava, and St. John's wort have calming properties to placate anxiety and stress, certain oils when used in baths, massaged on the body, or diffused by sprays in your home act as relaxants or mild stimulants.

Mind-Body Medicine and Body-Centered Therapies

Mind-body medicine uses techniques to try to influence the mind's ability to influence bodily function and symptoms by using such methods as meditation, prayer, mental healing, and dietary supplements (vitamins, minerals, herbs, and other botanicals). It may be that the brain and central nervous system influence immune, endocrine, and autonomic functioning, which is known to have an impact on health. There is ample evidence that mind-body interventions have positive effects on psychological functioning and quality of life, and may be helpful for patients coping with chronic illness.

Body-centered therapies include skilled use of hands, as in palpitation, chiropractic, which manipulates the spine, or osteopathic manipulation and massage. There are numerous types of massage including Swedish, shiatsu, and sports massage; each with its own theory on healing and soothing the body.

Energy Therapies

Energy therapies comprise the use of energy fields. There are two types: The first is biofield therapies, which apply pressure and/or manipulation to the body by running the hands in, or through, these fields. Examples include Reiki, therapeutic touch, qi gong. It has yet to be determined if these fields exist. The second type is bioelectromagnetic-based therapies that make use of pulsed fields, magnetic fields, and alternating-current or direct-current fields. These are invisible forces that surround all electrical apparatus. These therapies must be further studied to arrive at an understanding of if and how they work on the human mind and body.

Acupuncture

Acupuncture is a healing system developed in China more than 4,000 years ago. Acupuncture is a variety of techniques that stimulate points on the body using thin needles that pierce the skin and are then skillfully manipulated by a healer or by electrical means. Centuries ago, the Chinese identified hundreds of points on the body from which energy may be called for or liberated. An offshoot of acupuncture is acupressure, which uses the same points as in acupuncture, but in acupressure the points are stimulated with thumb and finger pressure and massage instead of using needles. Acupuncture is used to treat a large variety of complaints, such as weight, allergies, pain, respiratory, smoking, musculoskeletal, digestion, genital and gynecological problems, infertility, miscarriage, endometriosis, chronic fatigue, etc. It is effective in alleviating the physical symptoms of stress and anxiety, such as heart palpitations, headaches, insomnia, and neck and shoulder tension.

Acupuncture Practitioners

Finding a licensed acupuncturist has become relatively easy as more medical doctors are becoming trained in acupuncture and other CAM therapies. Some practitioners come from China and may not have a medical degree or are not licensed physicians in the United States. National trade associations may offer referrals to practitioners. A practitioner who is licensed and credentialed in a professional association may provide better care than one who is not. About forty states have established training standards for acupuncture certification, but states have varied requirements for obtaining a license. Although proper credentials are no surety of competency, they do indicate that the practitioner has met certain standards to treat patients through the use of acupuncture.

Treatment Cost/Insurance Coverage

A practitioner should inform you about the estimated number of treatments needed and how much each will cost. If this information is not provided, ask for it. Treatment may take place over a few days or for several weeks or more. Physician acupuncturists may charge more than nonphysician practitioners. Check with your insurer before starting treatment as to whether acupuncture will be covered as a treatment for your condition, and if so, to what extent.

Treatment Procedures

Ask about the treatment procedures that will be used and their likelihood of success for your condition or disease. It is vital that you make certain the acupuncturist uses a new set of disposable needles in a sealed package every time. The FDA requires the use of sterile, nontoxic needles that bear a labeling statement restricting their use to qualified practitioners.

The practitioner should also swab the puncture site with alcohol or another disinfectant before inserting the needle. During your first office visit be sure to tell the practitioner about all treatments or medications you are taking and all medical conditions you have. If you are worried about feeling pain, or afraid of needles, be sure to discuss this before you decide on treatment.

Aromatherapy and Bach Flower Remedies

Edward Bach, M.D., a homeopathic physician, claimed to have discovered the psychic healing properties of thirty-eight wild flowers. Bach believed that treating the person's personality characteristics, not the disease, would enhance healing. Bach believed that illness is a conflict between the person's need to use their energy to fulfill their lives (the "higher self"), and their personality which blocks and hampers them—thus creating distress and disease. He believed that flowers have a soul, or energy, akin to the human soul, and that the essences break down barriers that people have in living fully. He prepared essences of these plants and added water to make a drinkable mixture. Supporters of Bach remedies believe the essences are calming and provide the strength that allows individuals to cope with any situation.

The essences that are appropriate for helping stress and anxiety are: Aspen for anxiety, Cherry Plum for fear of being out of control, Crab Apple to boost low self-esteem, Elm to reduce stress, Mimulus for fears and phobias, Rock Rose for panic, Star of Bethlehem to heal trauma and shock.

Essential

Rescue Remedy is comprised of five essences: Star of Bethlehem for trauma, Rock Rose for fear, Impatiens for tension, Cherry Plum for fear of losing control, and Clematis for people whose mind drifts, is used to alleviate anxiety in humans and animals. The Rescue Remedy dose is four drops under the tongue when needed. Study of the controversial Bach flower therapy continues.

Aromatherapy was a term first used in the 1920s by Rene Maurice Gattefosse, a French chemist who used oils from trees, flowers, plants, and seeds to heal. The oils are thought to "balance the body" and provide relief for stress anxiety, insomnia, varicose veins, and various other illnesses and conditions. The oils are dispensed in small quantities and are made available in many forms: sprays, lotions, shampoos, creams, and bath potions. Diffusers should be included as they are one of the most popular methods of using these oils. Some oils are ingested and many are used in massage therapy. Menthol and eucalyptus oils are commonly used in over-the-counter medicines for colds.

Some of the most common oils' health claims include: bergamot helps calm anger; frankincense has a calming effect; jasmine lessens fear and lifts confidence; cypress promotes calm and quiets the nervous system; lavender alleviates stress; lime is a refreshing antidote to apathy, anxiety, or depression; neroli is considered an effective sedative oil; patchouli eases anxiety and depression; and sandalwood calms stress and fear. Researchers are studying the healing claims of aromatherapy, but much skepticism exists in the medical community. According to an estimate by *Health Foods Business*, the total of aromatherapy products sold through health-food stores in the United States was about $105 million in 1996.

📋 Fact

In 2000, Americans made an estimated 450 million visits to alternative health care practitioners—more than they made to primary care physicians. In 2000, people in the United States spent an estimated $2.5 billion on herbal remedies, including teas and supplements. These figures are expected to grow as the population ages, people live longer lives, and the popularity of CAM increases through the media and popular literature.

Ayurveda

Ayurveda is a holistic system of medicine that has been practiced in India for many thousands of years. The term Ayurveda is made up of two Sanskrit words: ayu, meaning life, and veda, which translates as knowledge of, or science; thus science of life. Ayurveda emphasizes disease prevention and proper hygiene and promotes a long healthy life. In Ayurveda the mind and body are considered to be interconnected—they are not viewed as the same thing. Together they form mind-body. There can be no mental health without physical health, and vice versa. Your whole life needs to be in harmony before you can enjoy true well-being. There have been published studies in medical literature that document reductions in stress and anxiety, cardiovascular disease, blood pressure, and cholesterol by individuals who practice the principles of Ayurveda.

Its followers believe that everything in the universe is made up of the five great elements, or building blocks: earth, water, fire, air, and ether. Earth is rock steady. Water is characterized by movement and change. Fire can transform matter and is considered a form without substance. Fire needs air to burn. This description is too "out there" and fundamentally meaningless without the following clarifier: It is a balance of these elements that creates health and an imbalance of these elements that creates disease. Air is what most animals on earth breathe. Air exists without form. Each person is seen as unique and when a health issue arises, the practitioner will advise changes in diet, use herbal supplements, cleansing the body of toxins, and suggest other lifestyle changes to effect healing. Ayurvedic medicine is taught in more than 100 colleges in India, and has been gaining popularity in the West. Ayurveda is a CAM alternative medical system.

Chiropractic

Chiropractic is a form of spinal manipulation, which is one of the oldest healing practices. Chiropractic is an alternative medical system and takes a different approach from conventional medicine in diagnosing, classifying, and treating medical problems. Conventional medicine is practiced by holders of M.D. (Doctor of Medicine) or D.O. (Doctor of Osteopathic Medicine) degrees and by their allied health professionals, such as physical therapists, psychologists, and registered nurses. Chiropractic training is a four-year academic program consisting of both classroom and clinical instruction. At least three years of preparatory college work are required for admission to chiropractic schools. Students who graduate receive the degree of Doctor of Chiropractic (D.C.) and are eligible to take state licensure board examinations in order to practice. Chiropractors are not licensed in any state to perform major surgery or prescribe drugs.

Coverage of chiropractic care by insurance plans is extensive. As of 2002, more than 50 percent of health maintenance organizations (HMOs), more than 75 percent of private health care plans, and all state workers' compensation systems covered chiropractic treatment. Chiropractors can bill Medicare, and over two dozen states cover chiropractic treatment under Medicaid.

Chiropractic Concepts

Most doctors of chiropractic, who are also called chiropractors or chiropractic physicians, use a type of hands-on therapy called manipulation, or adjustment, as their core clinical procedure. Some chiropractors do not use a hands-on approach. The basic concepts of chiropractic are as follows:

- The body has a powerful self-healing ability.
- The body's structure, primarily the spine, and its function are closely related, and this relationship affects health.
- Chiropractic therapy is given with the goals of normalizing this relationship between structure and function and assisting the body as it heals.

Several recent reviews on lower-back pain have noted that in most cases acute low-back pain gets better in several weeks, no matter what treatment is used. Often, the cause of back pain is unknown, and it varies greatly in terms of how people experience it and how professionals diagnose it. This makes back pain challenging to study.

Osteopathy

Osteopathy is considered an alternative medicine because in the United States, at least, it is considered a parallel discipline of conventional medicine as practiced by holders of M.D. (Doctor of Medicine) or D.O.(Doctor of Osteopathic Medicine) licenses. There are twenty colleges of osteopathic medicine in the United States Doctors of osteopathy may prescribe medicine. Osteopathic medicine specializes in diseases in the musculoskeletal system, believing especially that all of the body's systems work together and disorders in one system may affect function elsewhere in the body. Some osteopathic physicians practice osteopathic manipulation, a full-body system of hands-on techniques to reduce pain, restore function, and promote health. Osteopathic doctors also treat patients who require conventional care and medicine.

Conditions commonly treated by osteopathic physicians include back pain, neck pain, headaches, pain of arthritis, sports injuries, repetitive strains, and the stress and anxiety of patients with intermittent or chronic pain.

Dietary Supplements and Herbs

Federal law mandates that the term "dietary supplement" is considered a food and refers to products, other than tobacco, that are consumed.

These must contain a "dietary ingredient" intended to complement the diet. Dietary ingredients may include vitamins, minerals, herbs or other botanicals, amino acids, and substances such as enzymes, organ tissues, and metabolites. Dietary supplements are not considered drugs. It is recommended that before you begin taking dietary supplements, talk to your doctor. Many herbs and supplements may be harmful when combined with over-the-counter or prescription drugs.

There are many natural therapies and supplements available to relieve anxiety that have been used for centuries. Some of the most common natural herbs and supplements are:

- *Kava kava*: One of the main anti-anxiety herbs. It calms very quickly, is relaxing and mildly sedative. It is specific for anxiety, tension, stress, irritability, and insomnia. The USFDA has warned consumers that kava kava may be linked to serious liver injury, and that both kava kava and St. John's wort should not be used with medically prescribed anti-depressant drugs.
- *St. John's wort*: Is a gentle sedative, which affects the nervous system. It is specific for mild depression, anxiety, and tension.
- *Scullcap*: Relaxes and sedates the central nervous system. It is excellent for nervous tension.
- *Damiana*: A good nerve tonic, well known for its aphrodisiac properties.
- *Verbena*: Tonic promotes relaxation for nervous disorders and stress.
- *Chamomile*: Has been used for hundreds of years because of its rapid effect on circulation, digestion, and nerves. Used as a general tonic it relieves muscle pain and spasms, and insomnia.
- *Ginseng*: For thousands of years the Chinese have revered ginseng root because of its positive effect on physical and mental conditions. It is also believed to be an aphrodisiac.

Homeopathy and Naturopathy

Naturopathic physicians are trained in the use of a wide variety of natural therapeutics and generally do not prescribe pharmaceutical drugs. They utilize nutrition, herbs, flower essences, and promote general regard for the patient's psychic and somatic equilibrium. Naturopathic medicine promotes the theory that the body has a healing power that can restore itself to health. Naturopathic medicine is a CAM alternative medical system.

Dr. Samuel Hahnemann, a German physician and pharmacist, developed homeopathic medicine in the early 1800s. It is a holistic technique designed to treat the person as a whole being. It stresses the principle of similars; that is, treating like with like. Small, exceptionally reduced quantities of animal, vegetable, or mineral compounds are used to treat symptoms. Advocates of homeopathic medicine believe that these diluted extracts can be powerful cures for illness and disease. Examples of every day use of homeopathic remedies include treatments for the common cold and flu, hay fever, and digestive problems. Homeopathic medicine is a CAM alternate medical system.

Massage and Therapeutic Touch

Therapeutic touch (TT) is a controversial method in which the hands are used to "direct human energies to help or heal someone who is ill." It is using the hands without the hands ever touching the body of the patient. Its premise is that the "healing force of the therapist affects the patient's recovery; healing is promoted when the body's energies are in balance and, by passing their hands over the patient, healers can identify energy imbalances."

TT originated in the early 1970s by an R.N. and subsequent trials with the process have been largely by nurses in hospital settings. In the 1990s, nursing proponents of TT practiced it upon outpatients with MS in Pennsylvania hospitals. There was no sure response on the part of the patients as few could derive anything from the hands passing over their bodies. Except for the good feelings engendered when staff takes an interest in them, there was little to show that TT worked. That said, advocates of TT state that more than 100,000 people worldwide have been trained in the TT technique, including 45,000 health care professionals and that about half of those trained actually practice it. TT is sometimes used in conjunction with massage.

Massage is an ancient form of healing that has held its efficacy through thousands of years. The "laying on of hands" relieves pain, soothes the sleep-deprived, eases tight muscles, neck and shoulder cramps, and smoothes away anxiety and care. Massage therapists rub, stroke, knead, or slap various parts of the body to ease pain and heal. The benefits of massage are many and include:

- Relieves muscle aches and stiffness
- Improves circulation of blood
- Furthers skin toning
- Melts away stress
- Reduces anxiety
- Increases feeling of well-being

There are many types of massage, among them are: aromatherapy massage, which uses essential oils; and reflexology, in which the practitioner uses thumb and finger pressure on the reflex points of the feet. These points are presumed to represent other areas of the body. Asian-based systems of finger pressure on the points along "meridians" to balance energy are acupressure, shiatsu, and polarity. Relaxation massage, as the name indicates, is massage for relaxation and relief of tension and anxiety. Remedial massage is often used in tandem with medical intervention for injured muscles, tendons, and ligaments. Sports massage is a collection of many massage techniques to improve sports performance and relieve body stress from exertion.

If you decide to try massage as a way to alleviate your anxiety, make sure the massage therapist has studied at an accredited school, and has some experience working with your type of problem. Before you agree on a session, you will want to know how the technique is practiced, and what benefits you can expect. It is recommended that you ask to meet the therapist prior to your first session to see if you are comfortable with him or her.

Fact

The James Randi Educational Foundation offers $1 million to anyone who can show, under proper observing conditions, evidence of any paranormal, supernatural, or occult power or event. This is called the $1 Million Paranormal Challenge. To date, no one has collected the money.

Meditation and Yoga

Meditation quiets the mind. Meditation works through exercises, usually focusing on the breath or an object of attention such as a candle, and the repetition of soothing sounds called mantras. Prayer is very different from meditation. It is a practice that has a particular focus or intention and usually involves surrendering to a higher power and asking for guidance. Although it can be profoundly healing, it should be clearly distinguished from meditation. This sounds wonderful but is simply not the case. Meditation is a practice that helps us move into stillness, focus our awareness, and be with our experience in a loving and accepting way. It teaches us to slow down and be fully present in the moment. It also helps us to be present in our moment-to-moment daily life. Being fully present in the moment can, but does not necessarily, allow us to access deep relaxation and inner peace. In this way it can quiet the mind. But it does not cause troubling issues to recede. In fact, as we get quiet in meditation, it is a common occurrence for troubling issues to arise and disturb us. Through continued practice it becomes possible to allow both positive and negative, desirable and undesirable thoughts to simply pass through our field of awareness in a more neutral way. Deep relaxation is very healing. Metabolism, heart rate, and blood pressure slow, and muscle tension decreases.

Regular practice of meditation will help relieve anxiety by quieting the mind and allowing you to step away from disquieting thoughts.

All meditation practices have one thing in common: focusing the mind in the present moment and embracing all thoughts with equanimity. The purpose is never to distract the mind from unwanted thoughts. They do so by calling for concentration to one sound, one word, one image, or one's breath. When the mind is full of the healing properties of the chosen sound, or word, or image, or breath, its attention is riveted away from its cares; it will have achieved the beginning of the meditative process. There have been many investigative studies done on the efficacy of meditation, and we know from the results of these studies that meditation has both physiological and psychological benefits.

Yoga means "union" or "yoking" in Sanskrit. It is a mind/body/spirit discipline. It is the primary focus of Hinduism's varied religious activities. Though its geographical origin lies in India, its universal knowledge appeals to all peoples. There are many types of yoga. Four principal forms of yoga are: meditation (bhakti yoga), selfless service to others (karma yoga), practices for discrimination of truth and reality (jnana yoga), and meditational forms of exercise (hatha yoga, a part of raja yoga). Yoga aims to focus the individual on the true essence of reality through physical, mental, and spiritual activities, to achieve liberation and enlightenment. A man who successfully practices yoga is called a yogi, or yogin, a woman, yogini.

Essential

Meditation is an ancient discipline, though it was taken up by Western medicine only in recent years. It is safe and beneficial to everybody, and it alleviates and eases anxiety, stress, and many medical conditions. Meditation is known as a super stress buster. There are many types of meditation: Buddhist meditation, Zen meditation, TM (transcendental meditation), Taoist meditation, and, possibly the best known, is prayer.

Yoga offers one of the best means of self-improvement and realization of one's full potential. There are many clinical studies that show the effectiveness of yoga. It is a program immediately accessible to all without the fanfare of athletic equipment or special clothing and can be practiced by anyone regardless of age or physical condition. From a yogic perspective disease is caused by feelings of separation. Yoga is a discipline that joins together (yokes) the mind, body, and spirit so that we may experience our innate wholeness and create a space for healing. All it needs is commitment and a willingness to participate. Yoga works on the mind and the body at the same time as emphasizing their interdependence. Its techniques can be followed anywhere you are: in your home, office, on the factory floor, in an airplane, or while taking a stroll.

Fact

Yoga breathing balances the fight or flight response with the relaxation response. The fight or flight response is automatic—a sudden reaction without thinking, and one of the main aspects of it is the change in breathing to short, shallow, rapid breaths. You can actually stop the fight or flight from occurring and reduce anxiety by changing your breathing pattern to slow, deep yoga breathing. This breathing technique will engage the relaxation response, and put you in a calm state of mind.

The regularity of daily practice of relaxation and meditative exercises can make all the difference in how you feel if you suffer from anxiety. Imagine, you can actually take control of your anxiety, stop the fight or flight from occurring, and feel better in every aspect of your life. Yoga schools and other meditation organizations are popping up in towns all across the United States. Videos, audio recordings, and books also make these practices easy to do in the privacy of your own home.

CHAPTER 17

Self-Help Treatment for Anxiety

Controlling anxiety or even stopping it can sometimes be accomplished without the help of mental health professionals. Something as simple as changing how you breathe can stop the fight or flight from occurring, and help you cope with stressful situations. Many self-help treatments are available and can also be used in conjunction with other treatment you are receiving. Some techniques are very simple while others require more concentration and time. This chapter covers several self-help options.

Can I Help Myself?

Yes—you absolutely can help yourself deal with anxiety. Your initial step on the road to recovery is one of education. You want to learn as much as you can about the physiological process of anxiety, what the self-help techniques are, and what anxiety programs are available to you. You can help yourself to stop anxiety to the degree that you are willing and able to follow a healing program. There are many exercises and techniques that will help you recover from anxiety. They include: learning about anxiety, what it is and its physiological processes, diaphragmatic breathing, relaxation and progressive relaxation, desensitization, guided imagery, using yoga and meditation, etc.

With discipline and practice these techniques can stop a good percentage of your anxiety.

Your first stop should be to your family physician for a complete medical examination to determine if the root of your anxiety is caused by a physical disease or another medical condition. If you do not have a medical condition, then your physician may be able to give you information on how to set up a self-help program. Beginning a self-help program as either the only course of your healing program or in conjunction with medication and therapy is a proactive stance on your part and will help you take control of your anxiety instead of letting it control you. Helping yourself to heal will boost your confidence and build positive self-esteem.

Essential

It's advisable to join a support group if you are beginning a self-help regimen. There you can exchange experiences, not feel so isolated, and help one another learn how to cope with stress. One of the most beneficial advantages of a support group is that you know that you're not alone, and there are others who are suffering as you are.

Where to Find Information

You can find out what information is available to you by visiting your local library and asking the reference librarian what books, tapes, and other resources will meet your needs. Your librarian will also help you do a computer search. If you want to purchase the material for your program try and find it at the library first to see if the exercises and techniques are right for you. Or go to your local bookstore and spend time looking in the self-help section. Still not sure what to buy, make a list of the books that interest you and go to Amazon.com or Barnes and Noble.com and read the book reviews to help you with your decision.

The government's National Institute of Mental Health (NIMH) has Web sites devoted to all of the aspects of anxiety and the anxiety disorders, as well as written information that is free of charge. Other Web sites and organizations to check with are the National Center for Complementary and Alternative Medicine (NCCAM), and the Anxiety Disorders Association of America. To do an online search, enter "anxiety self-help" or other key words into search engines, such as Google.com or Yahoo.com. If you need assistance, ask your reference librarian. Support groups for anxiety are a wonderful resource. It is helpful to hear what steps others have taken to help themselves and what books, tapes, and programs have worked for them. There are many self-help programs to take advantage of either exclusively, or to meld, taking the best from each—as long as your application of the principles and practices continues in a methodical manner. These techniques will also be beneficial if you are taking medication for your symptoms and seeing a mental health clinician.

Breath Work

Unremitting anxiety can be very disturbing and frightening. One sure way to control the anxiety and eventually lose it completely is through the process of diaphragmatic breathing, also called yoga breath or belly breathing. It is a controlled pattern of breath work based on yoga principles. Yoga breath uses the diaphragm, not the chest, to slow the breathing process. Slow belly breathing can abort such anxiety extremes as panic attack, and modify other bouts of anxiety. This style of breathing slows mind and body and can transform you from being a nervous wreck into feeling calm and relaxed.

When you inhale, the diaphragm moves downward and when you exhale it moves upward. These movements influence all the organs in the body in a helpful effect that promotes better blood and lymph flow. When you're able to slow down, deepen and elongate the breath, your lungs will expand to take in more oxygen and release more carbon dioxide. The parasympathetic nervous system turns on to help keep you feeling relaxed and centered.

Breathing is both an involuntary and voluntary function. You breathe without thinking about it but can take control of your breathing patterns and engage the relaxation response by switching to diaphragmatic breathing, which is conscious application of a breathing technique. With practice you can learn how to control your physical, mental, and emotional functioning—just by breathing. The following are directions for diaphragmatic breathing:

1. Sit in a comfortable chair or lie down in a quiet place. Breathe only through your nose.
2. Begin with an exhalation. Breathe through your diaphragm, not your chest.
3. When you exhale, do so to a count of at least three. Your abdomen will contract.
4. When you inhale to a count of at least three, your abdomen will expand.
5. Keep your chest as still as possible, breathing should be slow, smooth, and quiet.
6. You want to focus on each breath as it goes in and out of your body.
7. If you lose the rhythm, or feel you're not getting enough air, stop, take a few regular breaths, and continue.

In the beginning, diaphragmatic breathing may be uncomfortable, but with practice it will become much easier. To be positive that you're breathing correctly, put one hand on your chest, which should show very little movement. Put the other hand on your belly, between the navel and ribs, and feel it pull in and push out when you exhale and inhale. You're aiming for a slow relaxed breath with no strain or effort. Practice while you are sitting, standing, and walking. Practice for three to five minutes at least three times a day while you are at home, work, and at play. For deeper relaxation, build up to a 1:2 ratio. Inhale to a count of 3 and exhale to a count of 6. Longer exhalations promote deeper relaxation.

Progressive Relaxation

Progressive relaxation (PR) is based on the principle that tensing your muscles, holding the tension for a short period of time, and then releasing the tension will result in the muscles being more relaxed.

Progressive relaxation was first used in the 1930s by a physiologist and psychologist Edmund Jacobsen who asserted that people could relax their anxious minds by relaxing their muscles in a methodical way. PR works because there's a relationship between emotional tension and muscle tension. If you are having an anxiety attack your muscles will automatically tense, and you will breathe rapidly and shallowly. But relaxing your body and muscles helps to loosen the mental grip of anxiety and engage the relaxation response.

Healing Effects of Progressive Relaxation

Progressive relaxation is one of the most effective ways to relax physically and mentally and is used to treat anxiety disorders and other mental disorders, insomnia, chronic pain syndromes, migraines, and many other ailments. There are both immediate effects and long-lasting ones, which include: feeling more relaxed generally, stopping the tension and worry associated with anticipatory anxiety, a decrease in panic attacks, being able to control your emotions and handle stress better, a boost in your confidence. If you practice regularly you will keep your body in a more relaxed state all the time and keep the "fight or flight" from occurring. Remember, you cannot be anxious and relaxed at the same time.

Guidelines for Progressive Relaxation

To reap the benefits of progressive relaxation it is best to follow the guidelines. These directions can be used for other self-help techniques that will be discussed later in the chapter such as guided imagery, yoga, and meditation. First record progressive relaxation script. Then set up a regular schedule for daily practice between fifteen to twenty minutes every day. You may either lie down or sit in a comfortable chair, wearing comfortable clothing. Make sure you are in a quiet place where you will not be disturbed. Don't have a full meal before practicing, it may put you to sleep. Breathe slowly and smoothly. Focus on the exercise, and when thoughts or worries intrude, gently refocus on the exercise.

How to Do Progressive Relaxation

Progressive relaxation takes practice to master, so when you first begin, don't give up because your success is going slowly. It'll take regular practice to arrive at a point where you can use it to quickly relax your whole body. The following is a short example of progressive relaxation. You can find scripts to record for progressive relaxation in self-help anxiety books. Scripts may run between twenty minutes to an hour.

1. Sit or lie down in a comfortable position and close your eyes.
2. Tense and relax one muscle group at a time. Start with your feet and slowly work up toward your head.
3. Tighten all the parts of your right leg, the shin calf muscle, knee, and thigh. Flex your right foot. Focus on the tension and hold it without strain. Hold it, hold it, now let go, release the tension and relax your right leg. Let all the tension flow out of your right leg.
4. Now, tighten all the parts of your left leg, the shin calf muscle, knee, and thigh. Flex your left foot. Focus on the tension and hold it without strain. Hold it, hold it, now let go, release the tension and relax your left leg. Let all the tension flow out of your left leg.
5. Now, in your minds eye, look at both your legs, and concentrate on letting even more tension go. Relax your feet, toes, shins, claves, and thighs. Keep breathing and relaxing and letting all the tension flow out of your legs.
6. Continue tensing and relaxing the rest of your body: abdomen, chest, arms, shoulders, neck, head, and face. When you have finished, take a moment to see how much more relaxed you are now than before the exercise. Mentally look over your body for muscle groups where tension remains.

While you are practicing diaphragmatic breathing you can add a technique of counting each breath to help you stay focused and keep anxious thoughts away. You can count "one" for an exhalation and "two" for an inhalation, or count each breath. When thoughts and worries enter your mind do not tense up—accept them and start counting and focusing on each breath.

Systematic Desensitization

Research has shown that a process of systematic desensitization has proven effective in the treatment of anxiety and phobias. In this scenario, events or episodes that have caused anxiety are brought up in imagination and coupled with a relaxation procedure. When this is repeated enough times in practice, the imagined event loses its power to generate anxiety. When you face the real event, you will find that it, has lost much of ability to frighten you.

 Fact

Systematic desensitization is a direct method that teaches you to respond to situations with an absence of fear, even though you may have held that fear for many years. You move at your own pace. Extensive studies of this method have shown that it does work, and better yet, the changes last.

The technique of systematic desensitization is a major method for eradicating fears. Systematic desensitization has changed the treatment of anxiety. In the evolution of the technique, eventual exposure to the object or situation in a relaxed and nonthreatening environment caused anxiety to lose much of its potency. Systematic desensitization has been shown to be effective for most anxiety-ridden phobias, but more so for specific phobias than for "free-floating" anxiety disorders, such as agoraphobia or social phobias. While initially created to be conducted by a psychologist or psychiatrist, systematic desensitization has been shown to be easily self-administered.

Guidelines for Systematic Desensitization

Desensitization is a technique that will be very effective in your anxiety program if you follow the guidelines and practice on a regular schedule. The first step is that you must be able to relax yourself quickly, on command by breathing techniques, and keep yourself relaxed as you face your fears. Other important features follow:

- You must be able to visualize what you are afraid of.
- You have created a hierarchy of your fear. For details on constructing your own desensitization program, see the Appendixes.
- You begin in fantasy desensitization—when you feel ready then you begin reality desensitization.
- Break down your fear into small manageable parts so you can do it gradually, in small increments, and build your confidence.

It is a good idea to chart your progress so you can see how far you've come. You may want to desensitize yourself by having a supportive family member or friend help you with the program. If you are working with a therapist, he or she can give you guidance and support, or you might have members of your anxiety therapy group give you a helping hand.

Guided Imagery

The mind influences the body. The mind uses images as its language. The images are processed not only visually but also through the sensations of taste, smell, sound, or a combination of two or more. For example, the smell of motor oil can evoke an image of an event that occurred more than fifty years ago; the sight and smell of a rose recalls a lost love. Perhaps your mind and body react to the smell of the oil with images of a serious automobile accident you were in, initiating the fight or flight response, even though the accident happened a long time ago. In the second event, the color of the rose and its perfume may make you flush with pleasure, or feel sad. Of the thousands of thoughts and images that daily flash through your mind, probably more than half of them are negative and many concern future worries.

You can learn to use guided imagery to help your body to heal itself, and get you where you want to be. Your imagination is a powerful force to help you battle tension, anxiety, and stress. Visualization controls and clarifies your imagination and is a technique that once learned, can be done wherever and whenever necessary. First you have to become aware of what your negative images are. Then you detail a positive mental image of yourself, or of yourself doing something you are afraid of, reaching an important goal, or anything you want to change from the negative to positive. Each time a negative image surfaces, mentally switch to a positive mental picture. See yourself as able to handle stress and anxiety in a calm manner. Picture yourself as taking home the blue ribbon, getting the job promotion you yearn for, or having the kinds of relationships you want.

Essential

The thoughts you have about things, people, and life affects the way you feel, act, and cope with life. If you dwell on the negative aspects of life more days than not, and feel saddened, anxious, or frightened by them, your attitudes about life will probably be mostly negative instead of positive.

Do your imagery every day. A good time to practice is in bed before you go to sleep. Practice diaphragmatic breathing to relax and help yourself become open to your positive mental images. You can couple visualizations with positive affirmations. Being able to see yourself as calm and able to handle your fears and anything in your life will, with time, become a part of your psyche, replace the negative pictures and thoughts you have about yourself, and ease your anxiety.

Positive Affirmations

Your self-esteem is vital to the way you handle yourself with people and in situations, and how you are looked upon. Affirmations are positive statements you say to yourself that state a fact that you believe about yourself, such as "I am a good person."

Affirmations are statements you can use to counter negative self-talk or the negative comments of others. And what you tell yourself, and your opinion of yourself, in relation to others and to the world around you contributes to your self-perception. If you say to yourself that you are powerless, can't change, are less worthy than others, stupid, or make other negative statements, then this will be your self-image and you will likely behave in ways to reinforce the negative image you have of yourself.

Fact

Affirmations have strong effects on the human psyche. If you're down on yourself most of the time, can't come up with anything in your favor, even the image you present to those around you will attest to that. It's hard to look happy and confident when you're feeling like a loser. But if you feel positive and confident about yourself, so will the world.

The Effectiveness of Affirmations

The power of affirmations, coupled with visualizations, are used by people seeking peak performance in athletics, business, and in roles of leadership. If you are anxious and have an anxiety disorder, you can also use affirmations to change your low self-esteem.

Many people with performance anxiety use affirmations coupled with guided imagery to reach their goals. For example, a runner visualizes the track, the distance when she will run, and the extra burst of speed necessary to win. She tells herself, "I will win!" All her training and will power has gone into getting her to this point. Affirmations are good techniques to add to your anxiety program and work very well when coupled with other relaxation techniques. Let's say you have panic disorder and are afraid to go into a shopping mall. You tell yourself that you just can't do it. If you go into the mall, you believe that you will have a panic attack and faint, vomit, go crazy, or die.

You can say an affirmation to yourself, "Yes, I am afraid to go into the mall, but I have the tools to calm myself when the anxiety increases." Or you can use affirmations like a mantra and repeat a short phrase over and over. "I will go into the mall." "I will go into the mall." "I will go into the mall."

Guidelines for Writing and Using Affirmations

It is important to know how to write and use affirmations. First, start all affirmations with an "I" statement, to make them personal and powerful. "I am a capable person." Keep statements in the present tense. Say "I will go into the mall today," instead of "Someday I will go into the mall." Avoid using negative words like "no," or "never." You must repeat, and/or write your affirmation as much as possible so it becomes internalized, becomes a true statement that you believe, not just a bunch of words without meaning. Couple your statement with guided imagery to make it more powerful and a fact of your life.

Stress Management

Though stress has a negative connotation, nonetheless it is part of normal daily life. Mild stress is a motivator enabling you to perform many of the tasks you've set out to do. However, if your stress level gets too high, social and medical problems may result. Dr. Hans Selye, one of the founding fathers of stress research, offered the view that stress is a "nonspecific response of the body to a demand." The definition most often used today is by Richard S. Lazarus: the "demands exceed the personal and social resources the individual is able to mobilize."

Stress is a product of everything we do and is different for each of us, so much so that what may be relaxing to one person may be stressful to another. For example, you may think nothing of a relaxing three-mile run during lunchtime, whereas your colleague may find that exertion stressful and avoid it. The management of stress is important so that we can remain calm in high pressure situations and avoid the hazards of long-term stress.

There are a number of ways to handle stress: confronting the cause of the stress, perhaps changing your surroundings, or minimizing the initial problem itself. Stress is a result of the way in which you interpret and react to events. Changing your perception of the situation will most likely lower stress. Accept the situation because there's little you can do about it and tell yourself you can hang tough. Accepting is taking control. While major changes cause stress, remember that less important stressors can build over time and cause tension and anxiety. Too much emotional stress will weaken the body's natural ability to heal itself, which may lead to illness and conditions like high blood pressure, ulcers, and heart disease. In the end, the best strategy for avoiding or mitigating stress is to slow down, learn how to relax, and make sure you have time for loved ones and leisure activities.

Spirituality

An additional aid to overcoming anxiety may be found in spirituality. This is the acceptance of a higher power with which you have a relationship. This relationship can give you inspiration, peace of mind, the feeling of joyfulness, and a deep satisfaction in knowing that there's direction you can count on. Of all the methods and techniques used in overcoming anxiety, a personal spiritual commitment is likely to reach the deepest in helping you to overcome the basic sense of fear or insecurity that underlies the various types of anxiety disorders. Whereas other methods work at different levels—body, feelings, mind, or behavior—spiritual awareness and growth can affect a transformation in your whole being. The more reliance and trust you develop in your higher power, the easier it becomes to deal without fear or worry with the inevitable challenges life brings. The resulting absence of anxiety is called peace of mind.

Journaling

Journaling is the process of writing down your thoughts, ideas, and innermost feelings and emotions. Keeping a journal is having a private diary where you can fully express yourself about anything you want to. You can write about yourself, your life, and others. It is a place where you can open your mind, heart, and soul and feel safe. You might want to write down your dreams and goals, and your journal may become a record of achievement. You may not think of yourself as a good writer—but you don't have to be. Your journal is just for you, so it does not matter how you write, no one is grading you on your grammar or spelling. Journaling allows you to spend time with yourself. It is a chance to get away from the stress of life, take a breather, and take time to find out about yourself on a deeper level—that's hard to do when you're running around feeling stressed and anxious.

 Fact

Research is being done on how journaling may heal both mind and body. A study in the Journal of the American Medical Association of people with rheumatoid arthritis and asthma showed that 47 percent of them improved after writing about traumatic events they had experienced. The control group wrote about mundane subjects and only 24 percent of them improved.

To use journaling to help you with your anxiety—try this. Write down anxious experiences you've had. Write down all of the thoughts, feelings, emotions, and symptoms that happened during this experience. Now look over what you have written. See if writing down what occurred helps you see the reality of the situation, which is hard to do when you're in the middle of an anxiety attack. Reading it in your journal may give you some distance from your anxiety. Then write down what relaxation and coping techniques you will use next time you are in the same situation. Writing down what you will do next time and what may help may build your confidence. Some people with anxiety use journaling to find the patterns when panic attacks will most likely occur.

Beginning a self-help program will require time, effort, education, and discipline. Discuss your plans with your physician before starting a program. Remember, practicing any of the self-help techniques will help you feel that you are taking control of your anxiety—and you will be. Seek help from professionals in the above areas to get yourself started.

CHAPTER 18

Diet, Vitamins, and Supplements

What you use to fuel your body has a major affect on your ability to handle stress and resulting anxiety. Certain foods and substances will increase anxiety, while others have been shown to decrease anxiety symptoms. For instance, research has shown that vitamin and mineral deficiencies create anxiety. This chapter discusses the importance nutrition plays in helping you to control anxiety, and simple ways you can use to tackle the condition on a daily basis.

The Effects of Food

You have probably heard the saying, "You are what you eat." Well, it's true. Since anxiety is a mind-body condition, its treatment requires a holistic approach. And nutrition is one of the most important aspects you need to examine if you suffer from anxiety. Researchers have been studying how food affects moods for decades. Studies show that certain foods and substances can decrease anxiety, while others will most likely increase it. Deficiencies in vitamins and minerals also affect mood, as do food additives, and food allergies. Experts in nutrition agree that poor nutrition will occur if your diet consists mainly of the following:

- Processed foods
- Foods high in sugar
- Fatty foods
- Food low in fiber
- Foods preserved with chemicals

If the above list of foods is the mainstay of your diet then it will be difficult for you to fight off daily stresses, and you will be at a higher risk to experience anxiety, and maybe develop an anxiety disorder. There is no doubt that anxiety and other mental conditions, like depression, are related to what kind of fuel you put into your body. These poor diet choices have a profound effect on your brain and emotions.

Sugar

Common white sugar is called a simple sugar and is made by processing juice from sugar cane or sugar beets. Sugar does not contain vitamins or minerals, and your body metabolizes sugar quickly, turning it into cholesterol and saturated fatty acids, while using up stored nutrients in your body. Simple sugars are absorbed into your bloodstream so quickly that the effects are almost immediate, producing a "sugar high," and raising glucose levels.

Sugar greatly increases the manufacture of adrenaline. A sugar overload may trigger the "fight or flight" response, with accompanying symptoms, such as rapid heartbeat, heart palpitations, jitteriness, and headaches. If you have an anxiety disorder, a diet high in sugar will most likely exacerbate your symptoms.

Fact

Simple sugars are hidden in many processed foods. The names of these sugars include: sucrose, brown sugar, corn syrup, dextrose, fructose, rice malt, maple syrup, molasses, and turbinado. You'll find sugar in breakfast cereals, breads, mayonnaise, ketchup, microwave meals, fast food, peanut butter, jarred sauces, yogurt, and hundreds of other food products. Start reading labels!

Salt

Salt is sodium chloride, a natural mineral found worldwide in seawater and underground salt deposits. Salt is a necessary ingredient for humans, animals, and even some plants. Salt has been used as a preservative and for pharmacological purposes since the Stone Age. In modern food processing, salt is used for many reasons, some of which include to stop the growth of microorganisms, to add taste to food, texture to bread, consistency to cheese, and for curing meats.

Too much salt will deplete your body of potassium, a mineral that aids in the functioning of the nervous system. It also raises blood pressure. Potassium has the job of making sure your cells and muscles function properly, it reduces blood pressure, and helps to balance the fluids in your body. When potassium becomes low the following symptoms may occur:

- Anxiety
- Fatigue
- Irregular heartbeat
- Thirst
- Chills

A number of conditions may occur with low potassium, which include vomiting, sweating, and diarrhea. High blood pressure medications will deplete your body of potassium. To keep potassium balanced, be sure to eat foods high in potassium, like: bananas, meats, fruits and vegetables, fish, and beans.

Foods Low in Fiber

Foods low in fiber have been processed in some way, for example, white bread is made from refined flour. Refined flour has had the bran removed, as well as all the nutrients and minerals contained in the whole food. If you have anxiety and want to increase your mind's and body's ability to handle stress, then you want to cut back on processed foods that are low in fiber, and increase your intake of high fiber foods. The American Heart Association and the National Cancer Institute both recommend you eat 25 grams of fiber daily. Whole foods do not contain sugar and simple carbohydrates and help keep the nervous system running at its peak, thereby avoiding poor nutrition, vitamin and mineral deficiencies, and mood swings.

Fiber can be found in fresh fruits and vegetables, whole grains, meats and seafood, dairy products, and legumes.

Research has shown that when you are under emotional stress, the levels of many vitamins and minerals in your body drop, which weakens your immune system, opening you up to developing physical and mental conditions. At these difficult times it is important to maintain a good diet, and adding whole high fiber foods will help keep your mental and physical reserves up and running.

Question

Does enriched white flour contain vitamins and minerals?
White flour is refined flour and the following percentages of vitamins and minerals have been removed: more than 60 percent of B vitamins, about 70 percent of minerals, and 80 percent of fiber, and almost 20 percent of protein. Some vitamins and minerals are added back to refined flour, but the percentages are way below that of whole grain.

What Is a High-Fat Diet?

Ours is a culture obsessed with weight and fat, and we are inundated with information about fat in our food. First, it's recommended that no fat or low fat will help us lose pounds and keep us healthy. Then we read about low-carb diets, because it is simple carbs that put the fat on, eating fats is okay. You need the real truth about fats to keep a healthy diet.

Fats are called lipids and are stored under your skin. Fats are an important part of a balanced diet. They help your body function well by keeping joints lubricated, provide chemicals needed by your body for proper development, help with absorption of fat-soluble vitamins (A, D, E, K), and are an energy source. And fats make food taste good. Fats are numerous; fatty acids and glycerol are naturally found in whole foods, such as eggs, nuts, and meats. Fats are also added to processed foods. There are two types of fat: saturated fats are solid, such as butter, margarine, and lard; and unsaturated fats are liquid, like vegetable and fish oils. Unsaturated fats can be partially saturated through hydrogenation, and turned into products like margarine.

Much research is being conducted on the connection between diets that are high in saturated fats and disease. Saturated fats have been linked to increased levels of fatty acids in the blood, which increase the risk for heart disease and for developing high cholesterol. High-fat diets may cause weight gain or obesity, which puts a strain on physical health, thereby making it more difficult to handle the mental and physical aspects of stress, which may lead to chronic anxiety or an anxiety disorder.

Reducing Fat in Your Diet

Many processed foods contain saturated fats, so read labels carefully. Experts suggest that the best advice on fats is as follows: fats should be no more than 30 percent of your diet, use unsaturated fats as much as possible, use processed foods sparingly, choose lean sources of protein like chicken, fish, and soy, trim excess fat off meats, skim soups, etc.

Preservatives and Additives

Thousands of chemicals are added to food to prolong shelf life, maintain texture of food, prevent spoilage, enhance flavor, and add nutritional value to processed foods. Additives include the following:

- *Preservatives*: Prevent spoilage and bacteria from developing, and oils from turning rancid.
- *Dyes/coloring*: Used to make food more attractive. Used in hundreds of foods, such as soft drinks, candy, and bread.
- *Sweeteners*: Includes saccharin, aspartame, sugar. Found in thousands of processed foods, such as desserts, soft drinks, and junk foods.

- *Flavor enhancers*: Almost all processed food contains flavor enhancers, which are called free glutamates, the most common being monosodium glutamate (MSG).
- *Vitamins and minerals*: Replace nutrients lost by processing; include vitamins, such as Vitamin D added to milk, and iodine added to table salt.
- *Emulsifiers, stabilizers, and thickeners*: Improve texture and consistency; include pectin and gelatin. Found in sauces and salad dressings.
- *Acids and alkalis*: Acids, such as citrus acid, are added to foods to increase tartness; alkalis decrease the acidity in foods.

Allergies to Preservatives

It is estimated that more than 75 percent of the Western world's diet is made up of processed foods. Many people have "reactions" to preservatives or additives, and decades of research have proven that food additives BHA, BHT, MSG, and nitrates are linked to a number of physical and mental conditions, which include: anxiety, depression, headaches/migraines, skin rashes, sleep disturbances, and hyperactivity in children. The additives' reactions range from mild rashes, to upset stomachs. More serious conditions can occur like asthma and irritable bowel syndrome (IBS). A life-threatening anaphylactic episode may occur that can cause symptoms such as anxiety, hives, nausea, stomach pain, and cardiac collapse.

Processed Foods

Modern food processing is done to preserve food, to kill bacteria, to extend the shelf life of certain food, to make it easier and faster to cook, and to be more digestible. Methods of food processing include:

- Cooking
- Canning
- Freezing
- Milling
- Drying
- Enriching

Critics of food processing point to the addition of chemicals, fat, salt, sugar, and the loss of important nutrients and fiber as problems in eating a diet of processed foods. For example, when whole grains are milled into breakfast cereal, the "bran and germ" are removed resulting in the loss of more than twenty essential vitamins and minerals. After milling, the cereal is enriched with less than five of the nutrients that were removed by the processing. Vegetables that are frozen and canned lose many of their nutrients but do retain some during the processing.

Since processing changes the whole food, the addition of excess fat, salt, and sugar to processed foods is done to improve taste and texture. For example, it is not uncommon to find from 600 to over 1000 milligrams of salt in one can of soup! And we have seen in previous pages that too much salt, sugar, and additives can lead to anxiety.

Essential

Eating processed foods sparingly or as part of a balanced diet is the key to fueling your brain so you can withstand stress and cope with anxiety. Nutritionists recommend that you eat as much fresh, whole food as possible. For example, use whole grains for some of your meals, eat fresh produce whenever possible, and choose low sodium processed foods.

How Poor Nutrition Affects the Brain

The brain is the center of all physical and mental functions. It is the seat of cognitive functioning, and emotions. The workings of the brain rely on neurotransmitters, which are the chemical messengers that relay messages from the brain to all other parts of the body, and keep it working right. A deficient diet will negatively affect the production of neurotransmitters, and cause brain function to be diminished, leading to a higher risk of anxiety, depression, and other mental conditions.

The human brain weighs on the average about two pounds, which is about 2 percent of body weight. But the brain needs lots of energy to function well, so it consumes 30 percent of your daily caloric intake. That is why if you starve your brain, you are negatively affecting your entire nervous system, and setting yourself up for anxiety, and other conditions. The foods that the brain needs are:

- Glucose
- Vitamins
- Minerals
- Other necessary chemicals

Besides eating a well balanced diet that will suit your needs, experts in nutrition recommend that you add vitamins and other supplements to keep your body and mind in top shape to withstand stress. A daily multiple vitamin may not be enough and you may want to confer with your physician about this, or get a referral to a nutritionist or other health care provider who specializes in anxiety and dietary concerns.

Fact

Of the more than 100 neurotransmitters in the brain, the healthy production of serotonin gives you a feeling of well-being, it calms your anxiety, and aids in helping you get to sleep. Dopamine and norepinephrine are responsible for intelligence, being able to think clearly, concentration, and memory.

Important Vitamins

Vitamins are organic food matter and are vital to proper brain functioning and overall health. They are found naturally in foods, and your body cannot manufacture most vitamins. Vitamins are obtained through food or vitamin supplements. Studies show that even subclinical deficiencies can affect your mental and physical condition and your ability to cope with stress. Some vitamins and minerals have also been found to play a particularly important role in the reduction of the symptoms of anxiety, and we have highlighted them below. Remember, before you start a vitamin and supplement regimen, check with your doctor.

Vitamin B1 (thiamine)

Vitamin B1 converts sugar into energy. If you have a deficiency of B1 you will feel mentally and physically fatigued, which can cause anxiety, loss of concentration, depression, insomnia, and stomach problems. Research shows that a diet of junk food that contains excess sugar will decrease levels of B1. Foods high in B1 are: oats, wheat, tuna, and salmon.

Vitamin B3 (niacin)

Vitamin B3 converts carbohydrates, proteins, and fats into energy. B3 is vital to healthy brain function and a balanced nervous system. Deficiencies in B3 cause irritability, agitation, and anxiety, and serious deficiencies can produce dementia. Foods high in B3 are: rice, chicken, turkey, and lamb.

Vitamin B6 (pyridoxine)

Vitamin B6 is essential for helping the nervous system function because it creates neurotransmitters. It also plays a role in healthy gums, blood cells, and antibodies. And, like the other B vitamins, it changes proteins, carbohydrates, and fats into energy. Foods high in B6 are: bananas, barley, chicken, turkey, avocados, and mangoes.

Vitamin B12 (cobalamin)

Vitamin B12 is critical for creating healthy red blood cells, and for the proper functioning of the nervous system. Necessary for the production of energy, it also plays an important role in memory and concentration. Foods: beef, lamb, shellfish, yogurt.

Vitamin C (ascorbic acid)

Vitamin C is essential for both healthy mind and body. Known as an antioxidant, it is also important to help you mentally cope with stress and reduce your risk for anxiety. Studies show that deficiencies are linked to the development of depression. Foods high in ascorbic acid are: citrus fruits.

Other Vitamins

Vitamin A is necessary for building healthy bones; biotin is water soluble and is necessary for other B vitamins to work well; water soluble B2 (riboflavin) converts fats, carbohydrates, and protein into energy and is vital for the production of antibodies and red blood cells; Vitamin D creates strong bones and teeth; Vitamin E is vital for circulation, healthy red blood cells, and muscles. Vitamin K is necessary for blood clotting.

Important Minerals

Minerals are nonorganic substances that are vital for physical and mental health, and they aid the assimilation of vitamins and help build new cells. There are sixty plus minerals in your body, which are found in your bones, muscle, tissue, blood, and cells in the nerves. Deficiencies in minerals can lead to mental problems, including anxiety and depression. Following are some of the minerals that are linked to coping with stress and anxiety.

Magnesium helps to relax muscles and calm nerves. It plays a role in helping your body absorb vitamins and keeps teeth healthy. Iron is vital for life, and the necessary production of hemoglobin, red blood corpuscles. Iron aids in physical growth, keeps fatigue at bay, and helps your body fight fatigue. Potassium helps neurotransmitters send messages to and from the brain. Zinc helps keep your body in a healthy state and plays a role in keeping your mental abilities sharp.

Choosing a Diet

There is no one healthy diet suited for everyone. How we react to and metabolize food is a unique experience. A food labeled as healthy may cause you to have an allergic reaction. For example, milk and dairy products may cause bloating and stomach upsets for people who are lactose intolerant.

You read earlier in the chapter that a diet based on processed foods or junk foods can either cause anxiety or worsen anxiety symptoms. Best choices are whole foods. You have also read how caffeine, nicotine, and other substances increase anxiety and may even contribute to the development of anxiety disorders. But there are certain foods that may actually calm you down. One of the most important tips about food and anxiety is to try and keep your blood sugar level throughout the day, because fluctuations can make you fatigued, irritable, and anxious. If you are not sure how to construct a food plan to help you decrease anxiety, at the end of the chapter we'll list professionals who can help you.

L. Essential

Researchers studying how food affects emotions found that carbo-hydrates elevate serotonin, because of the sugar and starch they contain. If you are feeling anxious, you might want to try eating a bowl of cereal or a baked potato before you grab a tranquilizer. Feel sluggish and fatigued? Then choose protein for a quick pick me up.

Chocolate

It is not uncommon for "chocolate cravings" to occur when your emotions are running high, and feeding your chocolate craving usually relaxes and calms body and mind. Some researchers believe that the craving is not just for the sugar, but for the sugar combined with fat. Chocolate contains the perfect combination, 50 percent each of fat and sugar along with phenylethylamine, an ingredient that causes endorphins to be released. Endorphins are pain-killing chemicals that occur naturally in your body and also produce feelings of pleasure and well-being. Chocolate can cause anxiety because of the caffeine content, but it also contains tryptophan, another chemical that creates calm feelings and sleepiness. Chocolate both stimulates and calms and is an antioxidant too. Experts suggest that a small amount of chocolate once in a while will not hurt you.

Bananas

Can eating a banana reduce anxiety? Musicians and other performers are using bananas to conquer performance anxiety. Many people claim that eating one or two bananas thirty minutes before a performance reduces the symptoms of stage fright, like shaky hands, heart palpitations, and the inability to concentrate. It is believed that bananas work to calm because they contain potassium and substances that act like beta-blockers. Bananas also have a thick creamy consistency, which may help to ease stomach problems caused by nerves. Since no research has been done on the banana phenomena, it is not known if bananas' calming affects are based on science or a placebo effect.

Fact

Performers commonly use grape juice to ease stage fright. Research shows that the juice increases the manufacture of dopamine, a neurotransmitter that transmits messages to areas of the brain that control movement, thought, and feelings of pleasure. Grapes are high in potassium and vitamins B1 and B2, and antioxidant properties.

Eating Guidelines

This section will help you set up a plan of action to use food to control or alleviate your anxiety through increasing the nutritional value of what you are eating and maintaining balanced blood sugar. Following these guidelines will likely make you feel more alert, energized, and able to handle life stressors. It is also recommended that you discuss any dietary changes with your doctor.

- Smaller and more frequent meals/snacks—eat something every two to three hours
- Eat adequate amounts of lean protein, like fish, poultry, yogurt, and soy

- Choose complex carbohydrates, like whole grains
- Fresh vegetables supply vitamins, minerals, and necessary roughage
- Eat fresh fruit instead of cakes, cookies, etc.
- Choose unsaturated fats like olive oil that support your immune system

To maintain levels of blood sugar, be sure to eat breakfast, and don't skip meals, balance carbohydrates with protein, reduce processed foods, alcohol and nicotine, become aware of foods that you cannot tolerate or are allergic to, and drink plenty of water. Try to make meals pleasurable and calm occasions, prepare foods you like that will satisfy your hunger, eat slowly, and enjoy your food.

Health Professionals Who Can Help

There are a number of health professionals who can help you set up a healthy food plan, and inform you about supplements and vitamins. Your family physician is a good place to start. Physicians will measure your height; weigh you; take down information on any allergies, intolerances, and dietary restrictions; and explain what and why changes may be necessary to your diet. Medical doctors will give you information about a good eating plan, and if you want more specific information, they may be able to make a referral to a dietary expert.

Dietitians and nutritionists plan nutrition and food programs and sometimes supervise meal preparations. They first assess your specific needs and educate you on healthy diets and dietary restrictions and modifications you may have to make. For example, restrictions in sweets if you are diabetic. Then they work with you to set up a program to meet your needs and keep you on track and will confer with other health care professionals who treat you.

📋 Fact

Dietitians and nutritionists require at least a bachelor's degree in nutrition and food, dietetics, or food service management. Dietetics is the science of food preparation and the planning of dietary programs. These professionals often work in institutions, like hospitals, but many have private practices and consult with individuals. Check with your state laws if dietitians and nutritionists require a license to practice.

Chiropractors treat health problems caused by dysfunctions of the nervous and muscular systems. They also emphasize adjustment of the skeletal system, especially the spine. The philosophy behind chiropractic medicine is that when these systems are compromised, the immune system is unable to fight off conditions and diseases. Chiropractors have a holistic view of health care and look at a person's general health, diet and exercise, environment, family history, and lifestyle. A bachelor's degree and four years of chiropractic college is required to practice.

Other professionals include physicians who practice homeopathic medicine, and registered nurses and other health care professionals with specialties in nutrition. You may also be able to get help from the numerous practitioners of "alternative" medicines and therapies. It is suggested that in addition to seeking professional nutritional help for controlling your anxiety, you educate yourself by reading as much as you can about how diet affects your moods. Go to your local library, bookstore, or check out online resources.

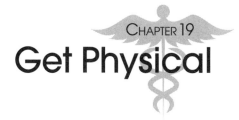

CHAPTER 19

Get Physical

Years of research shows that exercise is effective in helping reduce stress, tension, and anxiety. Exercising regularly is one aspect of a holistic treatment plan, and discussing this with your health care provider is recommended. There are numerous ways to fit exercise and physical activity into your schedule, and they don't all require paying for a gym membership or having a personal trainer. This chapter covers reasons why exercise is an effective method of dealing with anxiety, and some different methods to try.

Exercise, Stress, and Anxiety

If you are chronically stressed, anxious, depressed, and emotionally exhausted you are increasing the likelihood that your physical and mental health will be negatively affected. In previous chapters you learned that poor mental health is linked to heart disease, cancer, ulcers, high blood pressure, diabetes, and other ailments and conditions.

Many people live in an almost constant state of anxiety, with stress hormones spiking and dipping a little throughout the day. Then when they try to rest or sleep they are unable to do either, suffering from restless nights or even insomnia. Stress management guidelines list actions you can take to reduce stress and anxiety, and get on the road to all around mental and physical health, for example, eat regular balanced meals, and get enough sleep. On the top of the list is the suggestion to begin a program of regular physical exercise.

Alert

Before you begin to do any type of exercise it is important to have a complete medical exam by your family physician, especially if you have health problems. If you do begin a program educate yourself on the type of exercise you think will be fun so you will continue it on a regular basis. Start slowly on the level of your present physical condition.

Physical and Mental Well-Being

The connection between physical and mental health has been studied for decades, and the proof is in. The Perrier Survey of Fitness in America (1978) showed that people who committed to a regular exercise program reported being more relaxed, energetic, self-confident, and more productive in their lives. Researchers studying the effects of exercise on acute anxiety reported that the most common benefit of high intensity exercise was a reduction in anxiety. Numerous statistical analyses done during the 1990s all concluded that physical exercise significantly reduced anxiety. Regular exercise can relieve the worry and apprehension associated with anxiety. Becoming physically fit can help you tolerate stress much better, increase your ability to cope with life, and make you more confident, which increases self-worth and feelings of being capable in handling life problems.

So, how does physical exercise benefit psychological health? Experts studying the mind/body connection believe that the causes include: boost in self-confidence, taking time for yourself/being social, more oxygen to the brain, effect on neurotransmitters, and release of endorphins.

Exercise Boosts Self-Confidence

Studies show that when people start an exercise program and are able to maintain it, they experience a boost in confidence. Learning the exercise, sticking with it, seeing your proficiency increase each week, feeling yourself getting physically stronger, and enjoying the positive body changes (weight loss, development of muscle), all have a hand in your developing an increase in feelings of capability and self-worth.

Taking Your Time and Interacting Socially

Exercising allows you to turn away from the stressors in your life, at least for a little while. It is also something special you do for yourself. Exercising with others, or playing a sport may balance mood and emotions. Social interaction may take you out of your own problems for a while and having to socialize forces you to refocus on something besides your mood and symptoms.

 Fact

The U.S. Department of Health estimates that fewer than 30 percent of Americans exercise often enough to have a positive impact on their overall health. Research shows that hundreds of thousands of Americans die each year from conditions that could have been prevented by twenty to thirty minutes of exercise three times a week or more.

Benefits for Your Brain

Some researchers believe that exercise, especially aerobic exercise, increases the amount of oxygen to your brain. This increased oxygen elevates body temperature, which, in turn, enhances mood and eases depression and anxiety. More research is needed for proof and studies continue in this area.

Imbalances in the brain's neurotransmitters (serotonin, dopamine, and norepinephrine) are thought to be involved in psychological disorders such as anxiety disorders and depression. Research shows that vigorous exercise increases the level of these chemicals, and lifts mood and decreases stress.

Your Body's Natural Tranquilizers

In the 1970s, scientists located certain chemicals in the body called endogenous opioids that have the qualities of morphine. Endogenous opioids are divided into three groups: endorphins, enkephalins, and dynorphins. Research focused on the endorphin system because it aids in regulating pain awareness, blood pressure, and body temperature. Endorphins are associated with areas in the brain (the hypothalamus and limbic systems) that impact your emotions and behavior. During intense sustained exercise production of endorphins is increased by the pituitary gland, but it is unclear if the increase in endorphins can pass through the barriers surrounding the brain. Some researchers believe it does and that this increase is the cause of feelings of euphoria, or "runner's high" reported by athletes. Many experts state more research is needed to prove the theory.

Fact

The Surgeon General recommends thirty minutes of physical activity daily for overall health. That amount of physical exertion is necessary to burn the calories needed to reduce the risk of chronic disease such as heart disease and diabetes.

Other areas of study include experiments that suggest that sustained, modulated exercise that impacts the large muscles may activate opioid systems in the brain that trigger sensory nerves that go from the muscle to the brain. A number of studies do show that vigorous exercise somehow activates brain opioids, which increase ability to withstand pain and improve mood. Scientists continue to study the effects of endorphins on mood, emotions, and pain.

Researchers found that when you do aerobic exercise regularly your body builds up a tolerance to endorphins. As you increase the intensity and number of hours you exercise to produce the same endorphin release as when you first began to exercise, you will have to keep increasing the intensity and length of time. Since endorphins are similar to "opiates," exercise can become addictive, because some athletes begin to require the analgesic effects of endorphins, the "runners high."

Physical Activity: People Were Meant to Move

When you get stressed and anxious your body revs itself up in defense of danger and readies you to either stand and fight, or run away to fight another day. When the fight or flight kicks in, adrenaline and other stress hormones flood your body, chest breathing becomes rapid and shallow, and muscles tense as the body readies its defense for survival. This adaptive response to danger was designed to prepare you for vigorous movement. Intense battle or fleeing allows you to use the adrenaline and to utilize the tension in your muscles. Our ancestors lived much more active lives in general—walking as the major mode of transportation, hunting, farming, and other forms of manual labor that made up daily living helped to ease any build up of stress and the fight or flight. Today, most of us live sedentary lives and have to take time out of busy days to plan how we are going to fit exercise into our busy schedules. But our defense mechanism has not changed along with our culture. Our bodies are still revving up to protect from the stresses of daily life, but stress hormones and muscle tension have no way to be released, so they build up in your body.

Question

How can I lose weight?
You will need to burn off 3,500 calories more than you take in to lose one pound. The best way to do this is to eat fewer calories and be more active. About three-quarters of the energy you burn every day comes from what your body uses for its basic needs, such as sleeping, breathing, digesting food, and lounging.

If you do not presently participate in regular physical activity, think about a time when you exerted yourself physically—for example, cleaning your house or playing a sport. You may have felt bone tired after the physical exertion, but you were most likely much more relaxed and felt good mentally. If you do not engage in exercise regularly, you are missing out on one of the best ways to reduce stress and ease anxiety, and improve your health overall.

Guidelines for Exercise

Before you begin your exercise program, you will want to educate yourself about what different types of exercise are available to you, and what is best for you to start with depending on your age, health, and physical limitations. You'll need to figure out if working out in a gym or participating in a sport is what you want, or is working out at home the best plan. As always, the first step is to see your doctor if you have health concerns.

The following instructions will help you to set up a program that works and prevent injury:

- Do not exercise on a full stomach. Eat at least 1½ hours before exercising.
- Wear proper clothing for range of motion, weather conditions, etc.
- Warm-up before you begin with stretching, such as a range of motion exercises, and slowly start the exercise before moving into a higher intensity.
- Gradually work into a higher intensity for longer periods as your proficiency increases.
- Do not overdo it or you can hurt yourself or get exhausted.
- If you experience pain, nausea, dizziness, shortness of breath, or an irregular heart beat, stop at once and either go to your doctor or the nearest hospital.
- If an exercise hurts or is too difficult, move on to something easier.

- Always cool down gradually, bringing your heart rate down to its resting state.

Other tips to follow include: drink lots of water, do not hold your breath while exercising, cross train, and work out at least three times a week. If you are not sure how to begin you can find information at your local library or bookstore, or hire a personal trainer to create an individualized program for you.

Essential

Strength training builds up your endurance. It will help you fatigue less and decrease your chances of getting injured during other types of exercise. Strength training exercises include: situps, push-ups, working out with free weights, and using resistance machines like Nautilus equipment.

Aerobic Exercise

When you do aerobic exercise you are working your heart, lungs, and blood vessels, known as the cardiovascular system. No matter what you chose as your aerobic activity, it is rhythmic, repetitive, goes on for a period of time, and uses large muscle groups such as the ones in your legs, arms, and abdominals. The word aerobic means "with oxygen," and during your workout you will be increasing the level of oxygen to your muscles. Sustained aerobic exercise (sustained meaning for twenty minutes or more) results in a noticeable increase in respiration and heart rate. Examples of aerobic exercise include:

- Walking
- Jogging/running
- Swimming

- Bicycling
- Skating
- Skiing

Other types of aerobic exercises include: jumping rope, power walking, martial arts, tennis, racket ball, dancing, aerobic dance, and using aerobic machines such as treadmills, rowing machines, stair climbers, and stationery bicycles. Ideally, it's best to "cross train," that is, alternate between or among several exercises. Cross training helps reduce the possibility of the overuse of muscles and injuries and will keep you from getting bored. It is best to alternate between high impact exercises, like running or dancing, and tennis, and low or moderate impact exercises such as walking, swimming, and rowing. When stress has you upset and your anxiety is spiking, try running or a gentle jog, play tennis, go bowling, or take a short walk to release the pressure.

Aerobics in Your Daily Life

Some of you may have jobs that require manual labor and have aerobic activity during your workday. Landscapers, construction workers, farmers, etc., get to use their muscles and get their blood pumping. You can also put aerobics to work during the day at home; housecleaning, gardening, take the stairs two at a time, painting, and wallpapering all have aspects of aerobic activity in them. Think about what you do each day and see where you can make an activity have an aerobic component.

Exercise and Time

Though experts state, and research shows, that to get a good aerobic workout you need to do sustained activity for at least twenty minutes, many fitness experts believe that you should not watch the clock as much as set out to have fun. You can also get benefits from working out for short periods of time, for example, two or three times a day, ten minutes each time. Being too rigid about time may take the enjoyment out of exercise for you or make you feel that you have failed if you do not do at least twenty minutes—do what you can in the moment.

Benefits of Aerobic Exercise

There are many benefits to regular aerobic exercise, besides an improvement in mood and decrease in anxiety, and others, which we have discussed earlier in this chapter under general benefits to exercising. More benefits are an increase in energy and ability to ward off periods of fatigue. Exercise helps you to control weight, lower blood pressure, and reduce body fat. You will metabolize food better and feel a decrease in your compulsion to overeat. Your levels of HDL cholesterol, which lowers your risk for heart disease, will rise and your general health will improve, making you more confident and happy. You will reduce the risk of diseases such as cancer, and increase your mental agility.

Fact

The physiological changes due to exercise have been shown to keep the autonomic nervous system balanced so that your sympathetic nervous system that activates the fight or flight response is in tune with the parasympathetic nervous systems where the relaxation response is located. To be mentally balanced and centered these two nervous systems must be in sync.

Exercise and Your Heart

Throughout this book you have seen that anxiety is a mind/body condition. What physically affects you also has an impact on your mental health. You have also read in previous chapters how heart disease can be caused by chronic stress and the anxiety it brings, and that having heart disease is a real cause for anxiety. Keeping your heart healthy will of course benefit you physically, and will have a major impact on your mental health too.

Regular physical activity helps you enjoy life more fully. There is a growing recognition in the medical community and beyond of the importance of lifestyle and nutrition changes that can reduce the risks for coronary heart disease. There are four major risk factors for coronary heart disease: high blood pressure, smoking, high blood cholesterol, and sedentary lifestyle, or physical inactivity. Heavy smokers are two to four times more likely to have a heart attack than nonsmokers. The heart attack death rate among all smokers is 70 percent greater than among nonsmokers. People who are physically active are more likely to cut down or completely stop smoking than sedentary people.

 ## Alert

Coronary heart disease is the number one cause of death and disability in the United States for both men and women. Almost half a million people in this country die of coronary heart disease each year, and about half of these deaths are women. On average, almost three Americans will suffer a heart attack every minute of the day, that's half million attacks each year.

Blood Pressure

The higher your blood pressure, the greater your risk of developing heart disease or stroke. A blood pressure of 140/90 mmHg (millimeters of mercury) or greater is classified as high blood pressure. Regular physical activity can help reduce high blood pressure in some people. Exercise is thought to be a preventative solution and there is research that shows it may also prevent high blood pressure.

Blood Cholesterol

A blood cholesterol level of 240 mg/dl (milligrams per decaliter) or above is high and increases your risk of heart disease. A total blood cholesterol of under 200 mg/dl is desirable and usually puts you at a lower risk of heart disease. Different types of particles transport cholesterol in the blood. One of these particles is called high-density lipoprotein or HDL. HDL is considered "good" cholesterol because research has shown that high levels of HDL are linked with a lower risk of coronary artery disease. Regular moderate to vigorous physical activity is linked to an increased HDL level.

What Are the Risks in Exercising?

The most common risk in exercising is not preparing yourself properly to exercise and sustaining an injury to your muscles and joints. This is usually brought about by exercising too hard or for too long, particularly if you have been inactive for some time and are out of shape. Injuries due to exercise usually happen because you do not warm up and stretch adequately before beginning vigorous exercise. Getting injured in the beginning stages of an exercise program may cause you to drop out of exercising entirely. Being injured may increase your level of anxiety due to pain and added stress in being able to function on a daily basis.

Be sure you learn how to prepare yourself for aerobic exercise. If you have not gotten clearance from your physician and have a medical condition, exercise can cause you to become ill, or may exacerbate your condition, instead of help it. Another risk is heat exhaustion or heat stroke, which may occur on hot humid days. Both can be avoided by drinking enough liquids to replace those lost during exercise, keeping out of the sun, and limiting your physical activities to an air conditioned place.

Essential

If you experience the warning signs of chest pain, lightheadedness, fainting, and extreme breathlessness while you are exercising outside in warm/hot weather, these symptoms may be the beginning of heatstroke. Heatstroke can be fatal if not attended to immediately. These symptoms should never be ignored. Notify your doctor immediately or have someone call for you.

Stretching

Being limber and flexible by stretching the major muscle groups and strengthening the lower back is as important as aerobic fitness.

Keeping your muscles elastic will greatly enhance your performance in aerobic exercise. Weak back muscles make it difficult to move well, perform well, and feel good. Stretching will change that. Stretching also plays an important role in helping you reduce anxiety. A manifestation of anxiety is extreme body tension. Slowly stretching and loosening your muscles will help your body relax and will calm your nerves. Stretching your body will help you stretch your mind. Some of the benefits of stretching are that it:

- Relaxes your whole body
- Decreases muscle tension
- Prevents muscle strain and injury
- Increases stamina
- Improves posture
- Helps reduce mental tension and anxiety

Fact

Studies of older adults who have been on aerobic exercise programs found that the aerobic training increased many of their cognitive functions such as an increase in their reaction time and memory. Researchers believe that this occurs because exercise increases production of acetylcholine, a neurotransmitter in the brain involved in many mental functions.

Other benefits to stretching are: an increase in range of motion, promotes circulation, improves posture and balance, and increases concentration and focus. Stretching as soon as you get up in the morning will help you clear your mind, and signal your body that it is time to begin the day. Stretching at the end of the day before bedtime will relax your mind and will improve your sleep. Stretching also just feels good!

Stretching exercises should be done before an aerobic workout or other types of exercise. The only equipment you'll need is a mat for floor stretches. If you are unable to use the floor due to physical limitations, there are books and videos for chair stretches. Stretching has to be done slowly and carefully because overstretching can result in an injury that may take weeks or months to heal. Consider these tips:

- Do not strain or force the stretch.
- Do not bounce; gently hold the stretch for a few seconds.
- There should be no pain while stretching.
- Breathe normally.
- Don't hold your breath.
- Begin with easy stretches.

If you can find a personal trainer to help you begin a stretching program, do so. Or find books and videos on stretching at your local library or bookstore. If you are beginning a new exercise be sure to start with beginners stretches.

It is important to think about adding exercise to your anxiety program. Exercise will help you feel stronger, calmer, and more confident about yourself. It takes discipline to start and follow through on an exercise program. It takes time to make exercise part of your daily lifestyle. But research studies have shown that exercise is an important component in taking control of your anxiety. See your family physician as soon as possible and get cleared to begin an exercise regimen.

Chapter 20

Managing Life with an Anxiety Disorder

If you or a member of your family has an anxiety disorder, learning how to manage the problem while continuing on with daily life will go a long way toward facilitating the healing process. There are certain steps you need to take if you are the one suffering with anxiety, and other steps that must be taken if you are trying to help a family member with an anxiety condition. This chapter offers broad guidance on what to do with all the knowledge you've acquired thus far.

I Think I Have an Anxiety Disorder

There are some people whose lives are ruled by their fears and they are not aware of it. If anxiety began in childhood, or was an aspect of family life, then feeling afraid most of the time and experiencing symptoms of anxiety is just part of normal living. Maybe your parents or other family members had anxiety and you either had anxiety as a child or think you are having trouble with anxiety now. Perhaps you have experienced a number of major stressors in your life that overwhelmed you, and you feel stressed and anxious most of the time, but are not sure what to do. How do you tell your family if they don't know how you feel? Do you tell your boss and coworkers? Should you trust friends with this information? These are hard decisions to make.

It can be difficult to talk about how you feel and what symptoms you have, even with your family physician. So, the first step is to determine if you want to go to your family physician and discuss your problems. You might want to refer back to Chapter 2 and read over the common physical and mental symptoms of anxiety. If you have at least a few almost every day then you most likely need to seek treatment of some kind.

Steps to Take

Anxiety can make life miserable and stop you from living a satisfying and happy life. Facing the fact that you suffer from anxiety is the first step in overcoming it. Once you've done that, go to your family physician for a complete medical examination, and have the doctor do a battery of tests. After your doctor takes down your history and presenting symptoms, he or she will perform a series of medical tests to determine if you have a medical condition that might be causing your symptoms. An electrocardiogram (EEG), blood work, and other tests look for heart conditions, hyperthyroidism, and other conditions. If all tests are negative, your family physician may diagnose anxiety and either start you on an anxiety medication, or refer you to a psychiatrist, and/or counselor.

With a probable diagnosis of anxiety from your family physician, you have to decide if you want to begin a course of medication, or not. And if you do, would you rather your family physician monitor you, or would you prefer a referral to a psychiatrist for a medication evaluation. Getting insight into why you have an anxiety disorder and learning how to cope with and ease the symptoms will require counseling or therapy. You might want to go the self-help route, and that will take research and educating yourself.

Once you make decisions on the type of treatment you want, think about joining a therapy group or support group so you won't feel isolated. Having others who know how you feel assist and encourage you while you are healing, will help keep you on track and lift your spirits when you feel your treatment is not working.

Telling Family and Friends

Telling people about your anxiety may be a tough decision for you to make. Maybe you have been hiding the fact that you have agoraphobia, or are suffering from generalized anxiety disorder and it's getting in the way of your production at work. But telling family members and friends about your anxiety may help you feel less isolated. They may be able to give you needed support and help with your treatments, for example, have a trusted friend go out with you if you are working on a desensitization program facing your phobias.

Essential

Learn how to cope with your anxiety at home, work, and play. If you have a child, family member, or friend with anxiety find out the best ways to help them. Educate yourself about anxiety and the many treatments available.

Anxiety and Your Family

Maybe you have an anxiety disorder, or perhaps a member of your family is suffering. Either way, one thing is certain, anxiety affects the entire family. Sometimes, it takes years before the family realizes what is wrong. For example, there are cases where family members did not realize for years that the wife/mother had panic disorder with agoraphobia and did not leave home. How could that happen?

It happens because people with anxiety disorders are often ashamed about how they feel and behave. It's very difficult to explain to someone that going to the supermarket or driving more than two blocks from home will set off a panic attack and make you feel like you are going insane, or dying from a heart attack. You may be afraid that family members will think you are crazy, weird, weak, or lying. Unless a family member has experienced a panic attack, or has experience with agoraphobia, it is very difficult to explain why you can't go to the mall or drive on a highway.

An Example of Anxiety in the Family

Consider the following example of Laura's ongoing battle with anxiety:

Laura is in her forties. She has suffered from panic attacks since she was a child, and the symptoms have waxed and waned over the years. Her husband works and her role is to care for the house and children. For the last few years she has been having panic attacks in many situations and has become agoraphobic. Laura spends most of her time indoors and only goes out when accompanied by her husband. If she is required to go out alone, she makes up excuses not to go. Her parents live nearby and she relies on them to either go with her if her husband is working, or to do the task for her. As her children got older, she relied on them to either go out with her or to do her outside tasks. The relationship between Laura and her husband and children, and her parents is often strained because of her dependency and need to feel safe.

Laura never told a soul she had panic attacks until her teenage daughter began having panic attacks and didn't want to go to school—then she confessed to years of panic and told how she manipulated her environment to avoid going out alone. The daughter's diagnosis of panic disorder also opened up the same secret her mother had—that she too had panic disorder and also created a life of avoidance that no one was aware of.

Though Laura's refusal to go out alone and her heavy reliance on her husband, parents, and later her children was annoying, frustrating, and even caused a great deal of anger at times—the family viewed this as normal functioning. It was the daughter's diagnosis of panic disorder that showed them how unhealthy their lifestyle was.

Family Emotions

When there is anxiety in the family every member is impacted and has feelings about what is happening. Children whose parent has anxiety may be resentful, ashamed, angry, and disappointed if that parent cannot participate in the child's activities or family functions. Spouses may feel overwhelmed, frustrated, angry, ashamed, and sad if their partner cannot be an active family member, and the burden of the family falls on their shoulders. Parents may be worried, frustrated, and disappointed if their child is not an "A" student or is unpopular with peers and acts out every morning to avoid going to school.

Families are affected by anxiety because of the following:

- Family members feel helpless because they do not know how to help.
- The member with anxiety may not be able to participate in family outings/functions.
- Normal household routines may be disrupted.
- Family members may feel ashamed that their spouse/mother is acting abnormally.
- The person suffering may require special treatment causing jealousy and resentment.
- Family members may feel restricted by the person's inability to participate in life.

The Isolation of Anxiety

Anxiety disorders by their very nature isolate the person with the disorder, with feelings of shame, frustration, sadness, anger, and loneliness. Having a severe anxiety disorder may make you feel "different" than others. You believe that reaching out to people is hopeless because no one can possibly understand how you feel or what you experience on a daily basis.

Fact

People who have anxiety disorders often have a difficult time in their intimate relationships. One reason may be their coping mechanisms, which often include using drugs and alcohol—seen more often in men than women. Studies also show that people with mental disorders are at a high risk for divorce—about 50 percent of those in their first marriage get divorced compared to about 35 percent nationwide.

Family members may often be isolated and "sick," too, because of the restrictions imposed by the member with the disorder. Wives, husbands, and partners of people with anxiety disorders spend a lifetime trying to come up with explanations to friends and family why they cancel so often at the last minute to social events. Or trying to explain to their children why they never go away on vacation. If the family member with the anxiety disorder is the major bread winner, job and financial stability may be jeopardized due to excessive absenteeism, inability to perform adequately at work in stressful situations, and not being able to take promotions that require tasks that may cause anxiety and panic. Family members with anxiety may use drugs and alcohol to cope and isolate themselves and their family even more. Children with anxiety disorders often steer clear of friends, do poorly in school, and isolate themselves at home, maybe by spending too much time on the computer or watching TV.

Study in Anxiety

Tom had always suffered from anxiety, as did both his parents. He had panic attacks and also was generally anxious on most days, feeling jittery and nervous even while sitting in front of the TV after a day at work. Tom had no confidence in himself and each day was very difficult for him to get through. He had excelled at school somehow, and had a B.S. in economics and even managed to get an M.B.A. Tom was working for a finance company, and though he had difficulty concentrating, he did not think he was doing a good job and spent too much time double checking everything he did, his bosses liked his work. In the past year his anxiety had worsened, and he began having full-blown panic attacks at work when his boss promoted him to a position that required he lead weekly meetings and do company-wide presentations at least four times a year.

Tom was married and had two children. His wife worked part-time, and they relied on his salary to meet their expenses. As Toms' anxiety and panic increased, his job performance decreased. He began to get unsatisfactory performance reviews. Tom was never able to confide in his boss that he was having problems. Even his wife did not know the full extent of his anxiety—he was often moody, irritable, and did not want to do much when he wasn't working, but he could not bring himself to face his problems. Tom did not tell his wife how he felt or seek help for his anxiety until after he was let go from his job for poor job performance. His marriage was strained to the limit by that time, but he and his wife entered marital therapy. At the same time Tom began taking medication and was seeing a therapist for his anxiety.

Helping Family Members Cope

If you, or a family member, have an anxiety disorder, there are a number of things that can be done to ease family tension and at the same time help the family member who is suffering from the anxiety:

- Family members should learn all about the disorder—members are more likely to respond with understanding if they know what the effects of the disorder are on their loved one and themselves.
- Explain to the family that the member with anxiety cannot help how she or he responds when afraid—but that person is working on getting better.
- Have the family understand that recovering from an anxiety disorder may take a long time.
- The family needs to understand how treatment will work.
- Be flexible with household rules and schedules, but keep them as normal as possible.
- Do not show anger, frustration, or tease the person with anxiety.
- Do not try to "force" the person to do something that person is afraid of doing.
- Praise the person with anxiety for small achievements and accomplishments.

Family Therapy

Besides working on the suggestions above, it is important for family members to consider joining a support group or go into family therapy to work through the stress they feel, get support and understanding, and learn methods of coping and helping the member with anxiety. Family therapy will involve any family members that are important, and the therapist. You and your family will have a safe place to discuss how you feel and to understand each other's feelings and points of view. The therapist can also help you learn how to cope with and support a member of the family with anxiety. You can learn how to communicate better with each other, and how to express feelings and emotions in healthy ways.

Alert

It is important for family members to be supportive and understanding, but it is recommended that you do not "enable" avoidance behaviors. You do not want to force the person to do things they fear, but you don't have to make it easy. For example, if your family member always asks you to drive to the store, gently say something like, "No, I'm too tired. I'd rather you do it." Then praise the person for driving even though he was afraid.

Your Child and Anxiety

Children experience anxiety in their lives and can develop anxiety disorders, the same as adults. They may not have the insight that adults have about their feelings, and about what is happening to them, and their anxiety might manifest into different symptoms and behaviors than adults, but they are suffering just the same. Different types of events can trigger anxiety in children: divorce, beginning school, moving to a new house, death of a parent, and having to adjust to a new sibling. But like adult onset of anxiety, children may become anxious for no apparent reason. It is very difficult as a parent to watch your child suffer from anxiety and be unable to do anything to relieve their suffering. But you may be frustrated and angry, too, because of your child's behavior, for example, throwing a tantrum every time you want to go out and leave him with a babysitter. There are a number of anxiety disorders that children develop, and most times they need professional help.

L. Essential

If you are a parent and are concerned about your child's "fear," you may be asking the following questions: Is my child developing in an emotionally healthy way? Is my child on par with his peers intellectually? Or you may be questioning whether your child is exhibiting "abnormal" behavior. First, you have to determine if your child's fears are affecting him adversely at home, school, and at play.

The most common anxiety disorders in children ages six to nine are separation anxiety disorder and specific phobia. As they age, from age ten through adolescence, children prone to anxiety disorders are more apt to develop generalized anxiety disorder, and social anxiety disorder. It is difficult for parents to know for sure if their child's behavior is "normal," a passing phase, or something to be taken seriously that could lead to the development of a mental disorder.

When to Seek Professional Help for Your Child

It is frightening and upsetting to recognize that your child has an emotional problem and will need professional help. The first step for the parents is to discuss between them how they will approach their child about seeking help. A gentle but honest approach about how the child is feeling and what he or she is experiencing is the way to begin. Then, tell your child what your thoughts are about taking action: discussing the situation with teachers, guidance counselors, and your family physician. Allow your child to express their feelings, ideas, and concerns about your plans. Your child may feel frightened, ashamed, or relieved about consulting with professionals. Help your child to work through any feeling they have about getting treatment.

Symptoms in Children

Children share some of the same symptoms as adults with anxiety, but some symptoms are more common to children than adults and adolescents. As children grow into adolescence, their symptoms become the same as adults'. The behaviors and symptoms that demonstrate the need for professional help are:

Physical Symptoms of Anxiety:

- Racing heart/palpitations
- Dizzy spells
- Stomachaches
- Freezing with fear
- Crying
- Sweating/sweaty palms
- Tantrums
- Blushing

Behavioral Symptoms of Anxiety:

- Refusal to go to school
- Avoidance due to feelings of dread to feared things or situations
- Inability to socialize with peers
- Poor school performance
- Nightmares
- Irritability/disobedience

Children's Behaviors

Other marked behavioral changes include: the difficulty your child/adolescent has in coping with daily stressors, changes in eating and sleeping habits, and hyperactivity/extreme restlessness. Acting out behavior, such as drug and alcohol use; eating disorders; self-injurious behavior, such as "cutting"; and sexual acting out, signals emotional problems. Suicidal threats and threats to others should be taken seriously, and either immediately take your child to the nearest hospital, call a mental health professional, or contact the suicide hotline in the blue pages of your phone book.

When you are ready to seek professional help, first visit your family physician and have your doctor give your child a complete medical exam. Then get a referral to a child and adolescent psychiatrist or other mental health professional who specializes in working with children and anxiety. The specialist will provide information for you to help your child and, if a diagnosis is made, will set up a treatment plan with you that may include individual therapy for your child, family therapy, and medication.

Fact

The majority of adolescents who commit suicide have trouble handling stressful events and experiences, such as family problems, breaking up with a boyfriend/girlfriend, failing in school, and other major disappointments. Research shows that mental disturbances like anxiety disorders, depression, bipolar disorder, and drug and alcohol use are likely to accompany suicidal behavior.

Helping Your Anxious Child

There are many things you can do at home to help your child cope with his or her anxiety. Behaving a certain way with your child, and teaching your child exercises and techniques that they can use in fearful situations will help your child build their confidence and take control of the anxiety. The following are some measures you can take:

- Understand that your child's fear is real, even though it may seem trivial to you.
- Openly talk to your child about his or her feelings about being afraid to lessen the impact of the feared thing or situation.
- Never demean, tease, or put down your child for being afraid.
- Teach your child coping exercises and techniques, like diaphragmatic breathing, and changing negative self-talk to positive uplifting statements.

- When your child has learned coping techniques begin to gently guide him or her to face his or her fears.
- Educate yourself on the best way to help your child overcome and take control of his or her debilitating anxiety.

Involve Your Child in Her Treatment

Discuss with your child the ways in which she copes with fearful situations. Praise your child for trying to help herself, and work with her on improving her techniques or learning new ones. Have your child be part of her treatment plan to make her feel she has some control over her anxiety. For example, if she is afraid of going to school, discuss with her what techniques she thinks will work best, and where she wants to use them.

It is important to believe that your child has the capacity to overcome her anxiety. It is very difficult as a parent to watch your child struggling with her emotions and fears. But labeling your child as always fearful and scared may cause you to do things for your child that she can do herself. Take stock of how you feel and act when you are with your child. If you are lost about what to do, get professional help.

How to Handle Anxiety at Work

You may have anxiety at work, or have an anxiety disorder and are having problems coping with your emotions at work. Work and stress go hand in hand. Deadlines have to be met, you are overworked, prickly bosses have to be coped with, presentations have to be made, co-workers have to be handled. Whatever problems you have, if you suffer from chronic stress and anxiety at work, it can be a debilitating experience.

Become aware of your feelings and how you handle your emotions and interact with other people at work. If any of the following symptoms have become chronic, you may be suffering from work related anxiety, or have an anxiety disorder that is exacerbated by work:

- You feel that you cannot control your emotions, making you feel helpless.
- You suffer from loss of concentration and have difficulty remembering things.
- Your chronic anxiety stops you from having good personal relationships.
- You feel that you no longer function normally and this makes you afraid.
- Your appetite has changed: either you eat too much or have loss of appetite.
- You have trouble falling asleep or staying asleep.
- You have become irritable, edgy, and jittery every day.

Fact

Statistics show that more than 75 percent of the work force believe that they are under more stress than they were even a decade ago. Stress can lead to feelings of being overwhelmed and can lead to physical and mental conditions like burnout and anxiety disorders. Studies show that 27 percent or more of Americans feel that their job is the major source of their stress.

If you experience any of the above symptoms, either at work or due to work, and feel you cannot help yourself, go to the human relations department of your company, and ask for counseling if that is offered by your company. Or see your family physician and a private psychotherapist. It is important for you to be properly diagnosed so you can get the treatment you need.

Coping with Anxiety at Work

There are many coping strategies that will help you handle the stress and anxiety you feel at work, or to cope with having an anxiety disorder and having to go to work. The following recommendations will help you ease your anxiety at work. Learn how to breathe when the pressure is on; do diaphragmatic breathing that stops the fight or flight and engage the relaxation response. Learn how to prioritize tasks. Delegate tasks, or try to eliminate them from your job. When anxiety starts, breathe and stretch your body to reduce muscle tension. Learn how to do yoga stretches from your chair. Try to take time-outs during your workday—take a walk, listen to music, or read for a few minutes. Find supportive colleagues to blow off steam about work. Eat a healthy diet and exercise regularly to be able to ward off and cope with stress better.

Essential

If you have an anxiety disorder not related to your workplace, you will have to make a decision about telling your co-workers and boss about your anxiety. You want to think about the consequences if you tell them about your anxiety. Will it impact how co-workers and your boss view you? Will it stop you from being promoted? Will people make fun of you, or dismiss the seriousness of your condition? Before you tell, take your time to assess the situation.

Managing life with an anxiety disorder or helping a loved one with one is not easy. Anxiety affects every aspect of your life: family, friends, work, and leisure time. You do not have to go it alone though. It may be difficult to do but reaching out for professional help and telling family and friends can help you feel proactive about helping yourself. You won't feel so isolated and lonely, and you'll get love and support as you go through your treatment and reclaim your life.

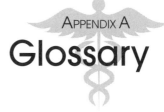

Glossary

adrenaline:
A stress hormone.

aerobic exercise:
Meaning "with oxygen," increases the levels of oxygen to muscles, also affects respiration and heart rate.

affirmations:
Affirmations are what you tell yourself to counter negative self-talk or the comments of others.

allergen:
Something, usually a protein, that causes an allergy.

amygdala:
In the brain, is involved with regulating emotions and storing memory.

anorexia nervosa:
Eating disorder featuring severe disturbances in eating patterns.

antidepressants:
Effective medication for anxiety related illnesses.

anxiety:
Uneasy feelings associated with apprehension from a real or perceived threat of imminent danger.

anxiety disorder:
A mental disturbance of thought or emotion that impairs normal functioning and creates psychic distress.

behavioral therapy:
Uses numerous techniques to change behavior.

beta-blockers:
An antihypertensive drug that works by "blocking" the effects of stress hormones, such as adrenaline, and easing the work of the heart.

binge eating:
A person goes through periods of uncontrollable binging and may or may not purge.

brain:
The brain is the center of all physical and mental functions. It is the seat of cognitive functioning and emotions.

bulimia nervosa:
Severe fear of gaining weight, person binges and then purges by vomiting or misuse of laxatives.

CAM therapy:
Complementary and alternative medicine utilizes a wide array of therapies outside of conventional medicine.

cardiovascular disease:
Affects arteries and veins that supply oxygen to the heart,

brain, and other crucial organs. Thought to be exacerbated by stress.

Cognitive Behavioral Therapy (CBT):
Therapy that seeks to decrease distorted thinking based on negative self-esteem. It is the preferred therapy today to treat panic disorders, phobias, and chronic anxiety.

cortisol:
A steroid hormone that positively affects stressful situations.

counseling:
Another word for talk therapy.

DSM-IV:
Diagnostic and Statistical Manual of Mental Disorders, now in its fourth edition. The standard guide for the mental health professional for diagnosing, setting up treatment plans, and aiding researchers.

depression:
A mental condition characterized by a pessimistic view of self, feelings of inadequacy, and a despondent inability to do anything.

desensitization program:
Desensitization program is simply exposure to situations and/or places that the individual has avoided.

diaphragmatic breathing:
Also called yoga breath or belly breathing. It is a controlled pattern of breath work based on yoga principles. Slow belly breathing can abort such anxiety extremes as panic attacks and bouts of severe anxiety.

dissociation:
Dissociation is a cognitive process whereby a person disconnects from his or her feelings, thoughts, memories, and sense of self.

distress:
One of two kinds of stress recognized by Dr. Hans Selye. It is disturbing, harmful, and causes psychic pain.

eclectic therapy:
Eclectic therapists use techniques from all schools of therapy tailored to the client's problems.

ego psychology:
Emphasis on strengthening the ego.

emotional stress:
Prolonged emotional stress can cause physical illnesses.

endorphins:
Endorphins are pain killing chemicals that occur naturally in your body and also produce feelings of pleasure and well-being.

eustress:
One of two kinds of stress recognized by Dr. Hans Selye in 1925. It is positive, such as falling in love.

exercise:
Regular exercise reduces anxiety and stress and will relieve many of the troubling symptoms of concern and worry.

existential psychotherapy:
The therapist helps the client face anxiety that arises from the reality of being alive and having to face death.

exposure therapy:
In phobia treatment, teaches gradual desensitization to the feared stimuli.

fear:
Though often given as a synonym for anxiety, fear is a reaction to a definable threat, whereas anxiety is not clearly defined.

fight or flight response:
A bodily survival defense mechanism against danger. The body prepares a survival reaction, called the "fight or flight."

gastroesophageal reflux disease (GERD):
Heartburn.

Gestalt psychotherapy:
Gestalt therapists focus on the interaction between client and therapist, rather than content. Believes that emotional disorders are caused by the client's unconscious needs: emotions, wishes, and obsessions.

group therapy:
Clients learn how to relate to others, see how others handle life situations, and feel support.

guided imagery:
Directed imagination used as treatment for anxiety disorders.

hippocampus:
In the brain, the hippocampus processes dangerous or traumatic experiences or events.

humanistic psychology:
Humanistic psychology seeks the goal of finding ways for the individual to achieve full potential.

hypertension:
High blood pressure.

hypnotherapy:
Developed by Anton Mesmer in the eighteenthth century, and refined by various practitioners since, these hypnotic techniques can put clients into a light to deep hypnotic state to help them overcome psychological or physical difficulties.

IBS:
Acronym for irritable bowel syndrome.

insulin:
A hormone that is needed to convert sugar and starch into energy.

meditation:
The effects of meditation have been shown to be associated with positive emotional states and improved immune function.

National Center for Complementary and Alternative Medicine (NCCAM):
Makes research grants and is the central depository for information on alternative therapies and botanicals.

National Institute of Mental Health (NIMH):
Main U.S. government information and research agency, conducts and supports research about mental health and mental disorders.

neurosis:
An unconscious mental condition that causes anxiety, conflicts in life, phobias, etc.
Neurosis is a term no longer used in the DSM-IV to define mental disorders.

neurotransmitters:
The workings of the brain rely on neurotransmitters, which are

the chemical messengers that relay messages from the brain to all other parts of the body, and keep it working right.

panic attack:
A panic attack is a sudden wave of paralyzing fear that begins without warning for no apparent reason, and seemingly without any way to stop it.

panic disorder:
A disorder in which the person suffers from severe panic attacks accompanied by distressing emotional and physical symptoms.

personality:
Personality is defined as characteristics that include attitudes, beliefs, thoughts, habits, emotions, and behaviors that make you unique.

phobias:
Phobias are extreme fears, irrational fears of an object or situation. Having to face this or even thinking about it can bring on a panic attack or a bout of severe anxiety.

progressive relaxation (PR):
Based on the principle that tensing your muscles, holding the tension for a short period of time, then releasing the tension will result in the muscles being more relaxed.

psychiatrist:
A medical doctor with a specialty in psychiatry.

psychoanalytic psychotherapy:
Based on the belief that thoughts, behaviors, and attitudes are controlled by unconscious drives and are not in our conscious control.

psychodynamic psychotherapy:
Emphasis on uncovering painful experiences and feelings to decrease symptoms.

psychological testing:
Tests that measure and evaluate human behavior.

psychopharmacology:
The positive response of mental disorders to medications sparked the growth of psychopharmacology.

psychologist:
Licensed after completing graduate work.

psychotherapy:
Helps individuals discover their capacity and capability to have a satisfying and productive life.

psychotropic drugs:
Medications used to treat emotional disorders and mental illnesses.

rational-emotive therapy:
Action-oriented therapy emphasizing clients' ability to think on their own.

self-talk:
What you say about yourself to yourself. Positive self-talk counters negative self-talk.

serotonin:
A brain chemical involved in regulating moods, promotes feelings of calm, relaxation, and sleepiness.

shell shock:
Name given to World War I mental breakdown, now called posttraumatic stress disorder.

short-term dynamic therapy (STDT):
Based on the principles of psychoanalytic psychotherapy but differs in the therapist's method of practice and goals.

social phobia:
Social phobia is an intense fear of embarrassing yourself in front of other people. Social phobics fear public speaking social situations like parties, and talking to authority figures like a boss.

social readjustment scale:
Also known as the Life Events Survey, predicts the likelihood of an individual getting physically ill or having mental health problems when faced with major life changes.

social worker:
Has studied clinical social work; licensed, many do psychotherapy.

stimulants:
Stimulants that affect the central nervous system are a broad based category of drugs whose characteristics produce feelings of euphoria, alertness, and a sense of well-being.

stress:
The body's physical response to events and circumstances.

stress management:
Stress is a product of everything we do. The management of stress is important so that in times of high pressure we can remain calm and avoid the hazards of long-term stress.

stretching:
Stretching helps to reduce the extreme body tension evident in anxiety.

sympathetic nervous system:
Produces the "fight or flight" response with the occurrence of stressful situations.

systematic desensitization:
Events or episodes that have caused anxiety are brought up in imagination, and coupled with a relaxation procedure. Proven effective in the treatment of anxiety and phobias.

talk therapy:
A dialogue between a person who is having problems, and a licensed mental health clinician.

telogen effuvium:
A loss of hair condition linked to chronic stress, depression, and sudden acute anxiety.

twenty-four-hour therapy:
A radical method that confronts clients with "reality" to help them develop self-sufficiency.

yoga:
Yoga aims to bridge mind, body, and spirit through exercise, breathing, and meditation.

Constructing a Systematic Desensitization Program

Systematic desensitization is an effective method of treating panic attacks, phobias, and avoidance behavior, first used by Dr. Joseph Wolpe in the 1950s. Wolpe found that people could overcome their avoidance behavior by learning how to relax deeply while facing their fears in stages. Two types of desensitization are used:

- Fantasy Desensitization: you "imagine or visualize" yourself with the feared thing, or in the feared situation, etc., while deeply relaxing your body. You practice in fantasy desensitization until the feared thing, place, person, etc., does not provoke an anxious reaction. In essence, you rehearse facing your fears in a safe place, and learn how to relax while doing so. When you feel ready, you move to reality desensitization.
- Reality Desensitization: now you face your fears up close and personal, but you do so with tools that will help you cope and handle the situation. By breaking down "big fears" into small pieces, and having rehearsed using fantasy desensitization, you likely will find that your anxiety level is manageable, and may have decreased.

Systematic desensitization is a method of treatment based on Pavlov's classical conditioning, also called associative learning. In classical conditioning two things, events, people, etc., are paired that causes you to associate one thing with the other. As an example, think of going to your dentist, and while sitting in the waiting room you hear the whine of the drill. If you have had painful experiences having your teeth filled, just hearing the sound of the drill might cause you to have an anxiety attack. Or if you have experienced panic attacks while shopping in a mall—then stepping into a mall, or even thinking about doing so may set off feelings of panic. In both cases you have been conditioned or sensitized to respond with anxiety.

Systematic desensitization is also called counter conditioning because it reverses the conditioning by reducing the level of anxiety to the feared stimulus, either the dentist or the mall. The reasons why counter conditioning works are: it is physiologically impossible to be anxious and relaxed at the same time, and you go at your own pace, one small step at a time allowing you to face your fears. The following are three necessary components to setting up your own desensitization program:

1. You must be able to relax yourself deeply and quickly with dia-phragmatic breathing and other techniques.
2. You have created a hierarchy of your fears.
3. You are able to visualize in detail your feared situations, event, people, etc.

A hierarchy of fears is created by breaking down your fears into the smallest steps possible (at least ten steps per hierarchy), and rating the steps from easiest to hardest. As you face and accomplish each small step, your confidence will grow and your anxiety will decrease. Create one hierarchy for each fear. Below is a sample hierarchy for someone who has panic attacks in a shopping mall:

1. Think about going to the mall.
2. Drive to mall, do not park, turn around and go home.
3. Drive to a mall, park, sit in car for five minutes, return home.
4. Drive to mall, park, get out, and walk to the front entrance of the mall. Do not enter the mall; return to your car and go home.
5. Go into the entrance of the mall and stand for a few minutes. Return to your car and go home.
6. Go into the mall and walk as far from the entrance as possible, then return home.
7. Go into the mall and go into one store. Stay for at least five minutes, then return home.
8. Go into two to three stores and buy something.
9. Go into as many stores as possible and buy a few items.
10. Walk the entire mall and go into as many stores as possible.
11. Shop and then get something to eat.

Additional Resources

This hierarchy can be worked through in fantasy desensitization first. You would imagine each step, and reduce your anxiety about it by breathing. You could also go right into reality desensitization either alone, or have a "buddy" go with you until your anxiety is decreased enough for you to work alone.

Guidelines for systematic desensitization are as follows:

- Work each step until you feel comfortable. Only then move to the next step.
- It is normal to experience setbacks—keep going.
- Do not set up a rigid time frame to be "cured." Work at your own pace.
- Positively reinforce yourself with something special as you complete each step.
- Plan to practice every day. But if you can't, don't be hard on yourself.
- Practice breathing and relaxing throughout the day so the techniques you are using work quickly in anxious situations.
- Chart your progress in a notebook/journal so you can see how far you've come.
- If you want to have a friend help, be sure you find someone who will listen to your needs.
- If you would rather have professional guidance, find a mental health clinician with experience in anxiety disorders.
- Celebrate what you are doing for yourself.

Sometimes a step on the hierarchy may elicit no anxiety. For example, if you are working the fantasy desensitization program and imagining driving to the mall does not cause a flutter, then either remove it from the hierarchy, or try to make the details of the scene more intense. On the other hand, if you have worked a step on your hierarchy many times and you still experience high anxiety, then either break the step down into smaller pieces, or rewrite your hierarchy so that the step comes later in the hierarchy.

Web Sites

About.com's Mental Health Web Site
A large resource of up-to-date information
http://mentalhealth.about.com

American Psychiatric Association (APA)
An extensive resource for information about mental illness and fact sheets about anxiety
www.psych.org

American Psychologist Association
Information on where to find a psychologist
http://helping.apa.org

Anxiety Disorders Association of America (ADAA)
A big helping hand for people with anxiety disorders
www.adaa.org

Anxiety Disorders: The Caregiver
A site devoted to support caregivers, family, and friends of people with anxiety disorders.
www.pacificcoast.net/~kstrong

Freedom From Fear
Site contains information on anxiety and depressive disorders
http://freedomfromfear.com

Mental Health Net
Covers a range of information about mental health issues, including anxiety disorders
http://mentalhelp.net

National Institute of Mental Health
A government site with much about anxiety disorders, and research in the field
www.nimh.nih.gov/HealthInformation/anxietymenu.cfm

Social Phobia/Social Anxiety Association
Web site contains information about support groups
www.socialphobia.org

Books

Bassett, Lucinda. *From Panic to Power.* (New York, NY: HarperCollins, 1995).

Bourne, Edmund J. *Coping with Anxiety.* (Oakland, CA: New Harbinger, 2003).

Bourne, Edmund J. *Healing Fear.* (Oakland, CA: New Harbinger Publications, 1998).

Bourne, Edmund J. *The Anxiety & Phobia Workbook.* (Oakland, CA: New Harbinger Publications, 2000).

Chansky, Tamar Ellsas. *Freeing Your Child from Anxiety.* (New York, NY: Broadway Books, 2004).

De Botton, Alain. *Status Anxiety.* (New York, NY: Pantheon Books, 2004).

Elliott, Charles H. and Smith, Laura L. *Overcoming Anxiety for Dummies.* (New York, NY: Wiley Pub., 2003).

Handly, Robert W. *Anxiety and Panic Attacks.* (New York, NY: Rawson Associates, 1985).

Hart, Archibald D. *The Anxiety Cure.* (Nashville, TN: Word Pub., 1999)

Luciani, Joseph J. *Self-Coaching.* (New York, NY: John Wiley & Sons, 2001).

Meyer, Joyce. *In Pursuit of Peace.* (New York, NY: Warner Faith, 2004).

Peurifoy, Reneau Z. *Anxiety, Phobias & Panic.* (New York, NY: Warner Books, 1995).

Index